Hypothalamic
Pituitary
Dysfunction

Registrars Office
RSCH .

Advances
in Reproductive
Endocrinology

VOLUME 6

Hypothalamic Pituitary Dysfunction

Edited by RW Shaw

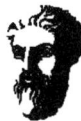

The Parthenon Publishing Group
International Publishers in Medicine, Science & Technology

| Casterton Hall, Carnforth, | One Blue Hill Plaza, Pearl River, |
| Lancs, LA6 2LA, UK | New York 10965, USA |

Published in the UK by
The Parthenon Publishing Group Limited
Casterton Hall, Carnforth,
Lancs, LA6 2LA, England

Published in the USA by
The Parthenon Publishing Group Inc.
One Blue Hill Plaza
PO Box 1564, Pearl River,
New York 10965, USA

British Library Cataloguing in Publication Data
Hypothalamic Pituitary Dysfunction. –
(Advances in Reproductive Endocrinology; Vol. 6)
I. Shaw, Robert W. II. Series
616.47

ISBN 1-85070-573-9

Library of Congress Cataloging-in-Publication Data
Hypothalamic pituitary dysfunction / edited by R.W. Shaw.
        p.   cm. — (Advances in reproductive endocrinology ; v. 6)
    Includes bibliographical references and index.
    ISBN 1-85070-573-9
    1. Endocrine gynecology — Congresses.   I. Shaw, Robert W.
(Robert Wayne)   II. Series.
    [DNLM: 1. Ovarian Diseases — physiopathology — congresses.
2. Pituitary Diseases — physiopathology — congresses.
3. Gonadotropins — physiology — congresses.   W1 AD83S v. 6 1994 /
WP 520 H998   1994]
RG159.H97   1994
618. 1—dc20
DNLM/DLC
for Library of Congress   94-17361
                                                                        CIP

Composition by Ryburn Publishing Services, Keele University, England
Printed and bound in Great Britain by
Butler and Tanner Ltd, Frome and London

Contents

List of principal contributors

D. H. Barlow
Nuffield Department of
   Obstetrics and Gynaecology
John Radcliffe Hospital
Maternity Department
Headington
Oxford OX3 9DU
UK

S. L. B. Duncan
Department of Obstetrics and
   Gynaecology
Jessop Hospital for Women
Sheffield S3 7RE
UK

P.-M. G. Bouloux
Department of Endocrinology
Royal Free Hospital School
   of Medicine
Pond Street
Hampstead
London NW3 2QG
UK

S. Franks
Department of Obstetrics and
   Gynaecology
St Mary's Hospital Medical School
London W2 1PG
UK

I. D. Cooke
University Department of
   Obstetrics and Gynaecology
Jessop Hospital for Women
Leavygreave Road
Sheffield S3 7RE
UK

S. M. Shalet
Department of Endocrinology
Christie Hospital NHS Trust
Wilmslow Road
Withington
Manchester M20 9BX
UK

R.W. Shaw
Department of Obstetrics and
  Gynaecology
University of Wales College of
  Medicine
Heath Park
Cardiff CF4 4XN
Wales
UK

M. de Swiet
Queen Charlotte's and Chelsea
  Hospital
Goldhawk Road
London W6 0XG
UK

M.C. White
Academic Department of
  Medicine
University of Hull
Kingston General Hospital
Beverley Road
Hull HU3 1UR
UK

Foreword

The isolation of gonadotrophin releasing hormone (GnRH) in 1971 and its subsequent synthesis gave endocrinologists the ability to further investigate and categorize the disorders of the hypothalamic–pituitary–gonadal axis. During the last 20 years our understanding of the mechanisms controlling GnRH secretion from the hypothalamus, as well as other feedback controls that act directly on the pituitary gonadotrophs, has been expanded. So too have other components which can influence reproductive function adversely such as surgery, radiotherapy and chemotherapy.

The application of the newer techniques of molecular biology is further allowing us to understand the intricate control mechanisms of this complex system as well as providing the tools to sub-categorize what until now have been broadly-grouped diagnostic categories of hypothalamic pituitary gonadal dysfunction. The adverse effects of prolonged deficiency of gonadotrophin secretion, particularly in young women, have also been appreciated and this has resulted in changes to our management approaches in these conditions. These were all aspects which were discussed in detail and are reported in this volume.

We were fortunate to be able to bring together a group of gynaecologists with specific interests in gynaecological endocrinology, as well as a group of physicians with reproductive endocrine interests. Together they contributed towards discussions of the basic science, clinical diagnosis and management of hypothalamic pituitary gonadal dysfunction in this meeting, the sixth in a series of international workshops on reproductive endocrinology. The meeting was held in Manchester in November 1993 and was kindly sponsored by Zeneca Pharma. This volume contains the contributions of the major speakers at that meeting and clarifies our current understanding and suggested management protocols for these varied, important and albeit uncommon conditions in gynaecological practice. It is hoped that this book will be of use to clinicians, both gynaecologists and endocrinologists, who deal with patients with hypothalamic pituitary gonadal dysfunction.

Professor Robert W. Shaw
Department of Obstetrics and Gynaecology
University of Wales College of Medicine
Cardiff

1

Mechanisms controlling gonadotrophin secretion

R. W. Shaw

INTRODUCTION

Gonadotrophin releasing hormone (GnRH) is a decapeptide secreted by neurones within the hypothalamus that stimulates synthesis and secretion of both luteinizing hormone (LH) and follicle stimulating hormone (FSH) from the pituitary gonadotroph cells. Both gonadotrophins are secreted by the same gonadotroph cells that constitute between 7 and 10% of the cells in the anterior pituitary. The secretion of GnRH is influenced by hypothalamic neurotransmitter substances, and ovarian steroid hormones, and higher CNS modulation later appears to be important in the aetiology of amenorrhoea and anovulation seen in some women under conditions of stress and following physical exercise and weight loss.

PATTERNS OF GnRH SECRETION

Studies of LH secretion in the female reveal that LH is released into the circulation in a series of pulses[1] and data suggest that each LH pulse results from the pulsatile release of GnRH by the hypothalamus. Although this assumption cannot be tested in humans, studies with sheep have supported this view, in that simultaneous measurement of GnRH in portal blood and LH in jugular venous blood have shown concordance between GnRH and LH pulses[2]. These data have been extrapolated to

1

imply that patterns of GnRH secretion in humans can be inferred from measurement of LH pulses in peripheral plasma.

This pulsatile secretion of GnRH is essential for the maintenance of normal gonadotrophin secretion and ovarian function. The crucial importance of the pulsatile nature of the GnRH stimulus was demonstrated in a series of studies in castrated monkeys that were rendered GnRH deficient due to destructive lesions in the hypothalamus[3]. These studies demonstrated that when GnRH was administered in a pulsatile manner, LH and FSH secretion was maintained at normal levels, whilst the administration of GnRH by continuous infusion resulted in an initial release of LH and FSH which was then followed by a fall in levels of serum gonadotrophins. These observations have been confirmed in women undergoing pulsatile administration of GnRH to induce ovulation[4].

The frequency of the pulsatile GnRH stimulus is also of great importance in determining normal gonadotrophin secretion. An increased frequency of pulses (to 2–3/h) reduces gonadotrophins in GnRH-deficient monkeys, whilst the effect is reversed by a return to a pulse frequency of 1/h. Likewise, a low frequency of GnRH stimulation (1 pulse every 3 h) failed to maintain serum LH concentration[5]. These studies demonstrate clearly the importance of the pulsatile GnRH stimulus for the maintenance of normal pituitary gonadotrophin secretion.

REGULATION OF GnRH SECRETION

Although GnRH is released in a pulsatile manner from isolated hypothalamus *in vitro*[6], this pattern of secretion can be modified by gonadal steroids and other neural signals. The most important modulators of GnRH secretion that are known are listed in Table 1.

Table 1 Modulators of GnRH secretion

Catecholamines	Inhibin
Dopamine	Oestradiol
Endogenous opioid peptides	Progesterone
Prolactin	Testosterone

2

Catecholamines

Noradrenaline has been shown to exert both inhibitory and stimulatory effects on LH secretion and its effects appear to be dependent on the presence of ovarian steroids, particularly oestradiol. In contrast, adrenalin does not alter LH secretion in ovariectomized animals but is more potent than noradrenaline in stimulating GnRH and LH release in steroid-primed rats. This suggests that adrenalin may be important in the steroid-induced increase in GnRH secretion that occurs at the time of the ovulatory LH surge. The role of dopamine in the regulation of GnRH secretion is less clear. The role of comparable mechanisms in the human female is uncertain since α-adrenergic receptor-blocking drugs (e.g. phentolamine) reduce serum LH in postmenopausal women and dopamine infusions also inhibit LH secretion in the female. These probably indicate a reduced GnRH release following such stimuli.

Endogenous opioid peptides

The endogenous opioid peptides endorphin, enkephalin and dynorphin may also play a role in the regulation of GnRH secretion. Opioid peptides inhibit GnRH secretion in humans, and long-acting enkephalin analogues inhibit LH secretion, whilst naloxone stimulates it[6]. Naloxone appears to act by increasing the frequency of GnRH secretion, and this action is most prominent during the luteal phase of the menstrual cycle, suggesting that endogenous opioid peptides are involved in steroid hormone regulation of GnRH secretion.

Oestradiol

Oestradiol can have an inhibitory action on GnRH secretion, as is demonstrated by observations that the concentration of GnRH in portal blood is increased following oophorectomy[7]. In addition, the frequency of LH pulses is increased in oophorectomized primates, suggesting that oestradiol inhibits GnRH secretion by slowing the frequency of this secretion. However, other conflicting evidence casts doubt on this simplified interpretation. The concentration of GnRH in portal blood is increased at the time of the LH surge[8] which occurs at a time of elevated plasma oestradiol levels. Additionally, the frequency of pulsatile LH secretion is increased during the late follicular phase of the menstrual cycle[9] and oestradiol can increase the frequency of LH pulses in ovariectomized sheep[10]. These data indicate that oestradiol can stimulate the frequency of GnRH secretion, and this action may depend upon a critical time–dose relationship of exposure of the hypothalamic GnRH secreting neurones to oestradiol.

Progesterone

Progesterone inhibits GnRH secretion by decreasing the frequency of GnRH release[11]. This effect of progesterone is seen as a reduced LH pulse frequency during the luteal phase of the menstrual cycle[9]; similarly, if progesterone is administered during the follicular phase of the cycle, LH pulse frequency is seen to slow[12]. Progesterone may exert this action by increasing the activity of hypothalamic opioid peptides.

Progesterone may also increase LH secretion, as demonstrated when progesterone is administered to oestrogen-replaced postmenopausal women, thereby inducing an LH surge[13]. This positive effect of progesterone requires the presence of oestradiol and is mediated in part by enhanced pituitary responses to GnRH (discussed below).

Prolactin

In physiological states of elevated prolactin concentrations (e.g. postpartum), LH secretion is suppressed, although pituitary responsiveness to exogenously administered GnRH is maintained, suggesting that elevated prolactin inhibits endogenous GnRH secretion.

The suppression of elevated serum prolactin after administration of dopamine agonists, such as bromocriptine, is associated with an increase in LH–pulse frequency and resumption of ovulatory menstrual cycles[14]. The mechanism by which prolactin inhibits GnRH secretion is uncertain but may involve increased dopamine turnover within the hypothalamus or increased hypothalamic opioid activity.

MECHANISMS OF GnRH ACTION

It is important to realize that GnRH is not only a releasing hormone, but that it has other important actions in the gonadotroph. A number of the components that have been studied are:

(1) Receptor binding;

(2) Signal transduction;

(3) Intracellular effector activation; and

(4) LH granule margination to the sub-plasmalemma zone of the cell.

Whether all of these actions of GnRH require the same transduction mechanism and effectors, or whether different effector molecules are responsible for each function, is not known. To date only one population of GnRH receptors sub-serving all of these actions has been described (Figure 1).

The GnRH receptor is located primarily in the limiting plasma membrane of the gonadotroph[15]. Attempts at pituitary GnRH receptor purification have proved difficult but available evidence indicates that it contains a glycosylated protein of about 60 kDa molecular weight and it has recently been cloned[16].

The availability of a GnRH radioreceptor assay has enabled studies on the overall relationship between GnRH receptors and serum and pituitary gonadotrophin concentrations in different hormonal environments. Such studies have demonstrated a positive correlation between GnRH receptors and serum gonadotrophins in two situations: after ovariectomy, and in the lactating rat – both situations believed to be associated with increased and decreased endogenous hypothalamic GnRH secretion, respectively. These studies have led to the hypothesis that GnRH, by a direct action on gonadotrophs, is the major hormonal determinant of the pituitary GnRH receptor content. (For a review, see reference 17). Direct evidence that GnRH upregulates its own receptors was provided from *in vivo* studies of chronic pulsatile GnRH treatment in animals with absent GnRH secretions[18]. These data have indicated that GnRH is one of the few hormones that has been shown to induce its own receptors and that these may be a prerequisite for (or at least part of) an appropriate physiological response to altered hormonal milieu.

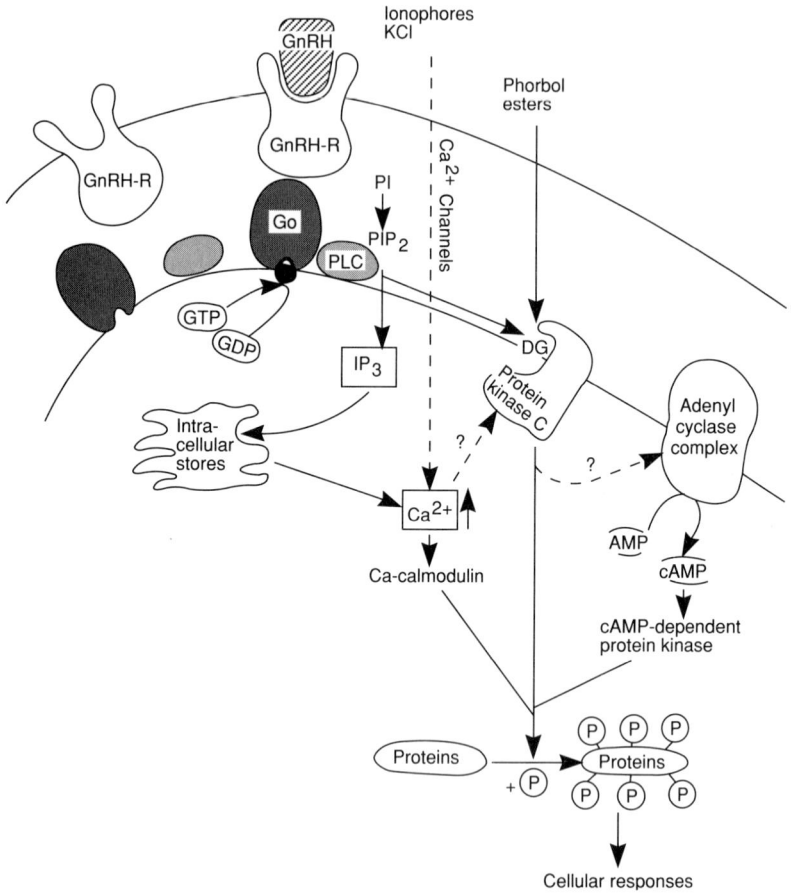

Figure 1 Schematic representation of gonadotrophin releasing hormone receptor (GnRH-R) signal transduction. cAMP = cyclic adenosine monophosphate; DG = diacylglycerol; GDP = guanosine diphosphate; GTP = guanosine triphosphate; Go = GTP binding protein; IP_3 = inositol phosphate; PI = phosphatidylinositol; PIP_2 = phosphatidylinositol-4,5-bisphosphate; PLC = phospholipase C; P = phosphate group. (Reproduced with permission from ref. 32)

Regulation by oestrogen

An enhanced pituitary sensitivity to GnRH in mammals is observed prior to the preovulatory LH surge and is dependent upon increasing ovarian oestrogen production. Twofold to threefold increases in GnRH receptors have been demonstrated to occur at the time of rising serum oestradiol concentrations in rats[19]. In addition, exogenous oestrogen treatment to ovariectomized monkeys produces a GnRH receptor increase coincident with the oestrogen-induced LH surge[20].

These data point to the important role for oestrogen in the induction of GnRH receptors during the process of the LH surge induction. Rising serum oestradiol concentrations during the days that precede the LH surge induce GnRH receptors, enabling the pituitary to respond to sub-threshhold concentrations of GnRH in the portal blood. This has the effect of generating a continuous LH secretion that accumulates to produce the high preovulatory levels. Such a mechanism could explain the LH surge, without the need to invoke an increase in endogenous GnRH pulse frequency or amplitude.

GONADOTROPH DESENSITIZATION

Refractoriness of cells to stimulation by a homologous ligand after a preceding exposure to that ligand is a common biological phenomenon that has perhaps evolved as a protective measure against repetitive activation. This phenomenon has been well characterized for surface-active peptide hormones. Persistent refractoriness or 'desensitization' can be induced by prolonged and continuous exposure to the ligand. Such a situation applies to GnRH and gonadotrophs. Although gonadotrophin desensitization (or downregulation) can be achieved with native GnRH, it is much more readily seen with those highly potent super-agonists which have been developed which have high receptor affinity and a prolonged biological half-life. Using a superactive agonist in the rat, pituitary desensitization was induced by continuous infusion over a number of days with a marked (80%) reduction in subsequent ligand binding. A proportion of this is accounted for by the occupancy of receptors by the exogenous hormone (60%), with true receptor loss or downregulation accounting for some 40% of the decline[21]. Thus desensitization is only partially explained by receptor loss, since many receptors are occupied by the agonist whilst serum LH levels are found to be dramatically reduced. This suggests there must be additional mechanisms involved – for example the disruption of post-receptor transductor/effector mechanisms.

This desensitization is not dependent upon LH release since it occurs in the absence of extracellular calcium which prevents secretion of LH. Likewise, receptor internalization is not involved[22]. However, desensitization is receptor-mediated because other LH stimulatory agents (e.g. calcium ionophores, depolarization) do not reduce subsequent responses to GnRH. Thus the nature of the post-receptor lesion is unclear. It appears to be complex, consisting of at least three components: receptor downregulation; the uncoupling of remaining GnRH receptors from effector signals; and the inhibition of hormone synthesis.

SIGNAL TRANSDUCTION AND INTRACELLULAR EFFECTS

Much has been learnt of the cellular events involved in serial transduction and the generation of intracellular effectors following GnRH receptor activation. A schematic chain of events is summarized in Figure 1. Within seconds of GnRH receptor activation, intracellular free calcium concentrations rise[23], probably as a result of the immobilization of intracellular stores of calcium. A sustained release of LH is also calcium-dependent, originating from extracellular calcium entering through receptor-regulated voltage-dependent calcium channels[23]. The initial mobilization of intracellular calcium is occasioned by inositol trisphosphate which accumulates rapidly as the result of receptor activation of the membrane-bound enzyme phospholipase C which breaks down membrane polyphosphoinositides[24]. Diacylglycerol is a second product of phospholipase C action and activates the potent phosphorylating enzyme protein kinase C. The activation of protein kinase C induces a submaximal LH release, but when calcium is increased simultaneously, maximum release occurs. The roles of adenylcyclase, cyclic adenosine monophosphate (cAMP), receptor activation and the intracellular effect on these mechanisms are still unclear.

In addition to its action as a releaser of LH and FSH, it is now clear that GnRH acts as a trophic hormone. It seems likely that these trophic actions are exerted at the nuclear level by the stimulation of specific gene transcription. Support for this theory is provided by animal studies which show increased gonadotrophin subunit mRNA levels after castration[25]. As well as its actions in the early steps of LH biosynthesis, GnRH also stimulates the glycosylation of mRNA subunits, hence influencing the bioactivity of the hormone production which is enhanced by oestradiol[26].

MODULATION OF GONADOTROPHIN RESPONSES TO GnRH

Current evidence indicates that oestradiol and progesterone are the most important hormones involved in the regulation of gonodotroph responsiveness to GnRH. However, other ovarian compounds such as inhibin, and pituitary hormones such as prolactin or adrenal steroids, may have a role in modulating this responsiveness.

Oestradiol

Pituitary responsiveness to a fixed dose of exogenous GnRH varies throughout the menstrual cycle. The greatest LH release is observed during the periovulatory period with the next highest levels occurring in the luteal phase. Whilst there is marked individual variation throughout a single menstrual cycle, there is a positive correlation within individuals between LH peak response to exogenous GnRH and circulating oestradiol levels[27] (Figure 2).

Studies using single or multiple injections of GnRH have shown that both the inhibitory and stimulatory effects of oestradiol are exerted on the pituitary gonadotroph. Following oestradiol administration to normal women, LH responses to GnRH are suppressed during the first 36 h but augmented responses are seen after 48 h and persist for several days [28].

The time-course of the positive and negative feedback effects of oestradiol depend both upon the species studied and the dose of oestradiol. The temporal relationships have been closly studied, at least in sheep, and are demonstrated in Figure 3. Oestradiol initially inhibits LH release in response to each GnRH pulse but the subseqent LH responses are augmented and mean plasma LH concentration increased. In contrast to the effects on LH, oestradiol exerts an inhibitory action on FSH release.

Progesterone

Progesterone can also augment gonadotrophin responses to GnRH but this action is only seen after previous exposure to oestradiol. This was evident when responsiveness to GnRH was tested in the early follicular phase of the cycle with low endogenous oestrogen levels in which progesterone pretreatment produced only a small increase in LH increments following

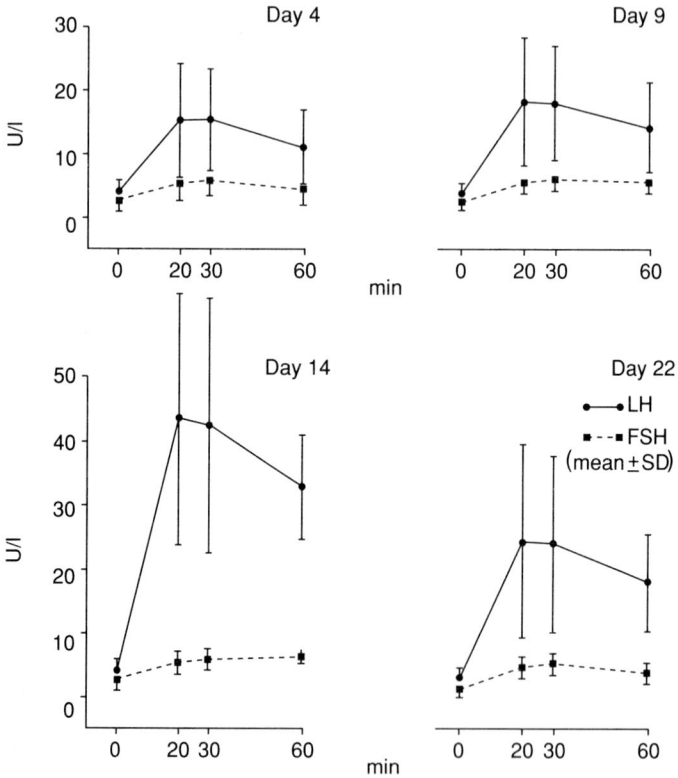

Figure 2 Variation in pituitary responsiveness to exogenous GnRH (100 µg, intravenously) at different stages of the same menstrual cycle in a group of regularly menstruating females. (Modified from ref. 27)

exogenous GnRH administration. This is in contrast to the marked augmentation effects observed in the mid-follicular phase of the cycle (days 8–10) when endogenous oestradiol levels are much higher. In this situation progesterone treatment led to marked increases in pituitary responsiveness following progesterone pretreatment. Such data suggest that progesterone acts synergistically with oestrogen to augment gonadotrophin responsiveness of GnRH[29]. The combined effects of these steroids is a crucial factor in the production of the midcycle LH and FSH surge, with progesterone augmenting and prolonging the positive feedback effects of oestradiol.

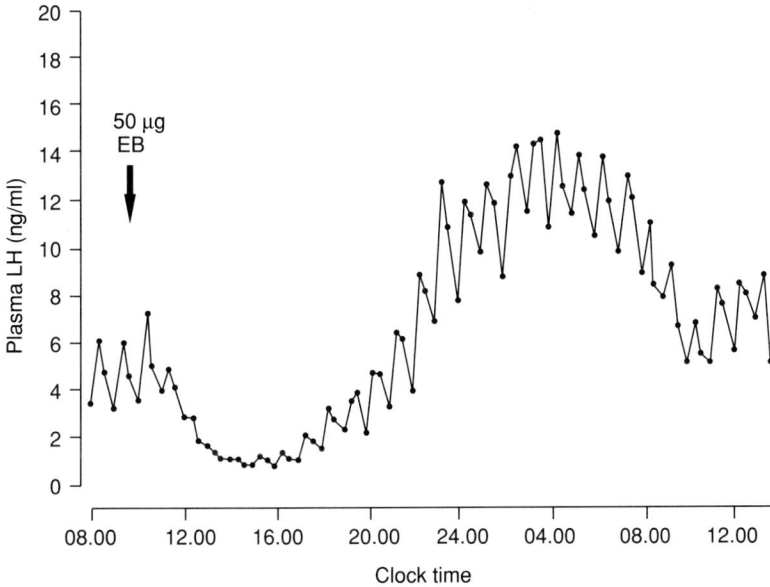

Figure 3 The inhibitory and stimulatory effects of oestradiol on LH responsiveness to GnRH in ovariectomized ewes with surgical disconnection of the hypothalamus from the pituitary. GnRH pulses of 500 ng were administered every 1 h, and 50 μg of oestradiol benzoate (EB) as indicated. (From ref. 33, with permission from S. Karger AG, Basel)

Prolactin

The main effects of prolactin on LH and FSH secretion appear to be exerted by the inhibition of GnRH secretion. However, data from rat studies suggest that marked or prolonged elevation of prolactin may inhibit the pituitary response to GnRH *in vivo* and contribute to the low levels of gonadotrophin secretion observed in hyperprolactinaemic states[30].

Inhibin

Follicular fluid appears to contain substances other than steroid hormones that play a role in the regulation of gonadotrophin secretion. Following treatment of follicular fluid with activated charcoal to remove steroids, it has been shown that such fluid can selectively inhibit FSH secretion in female rats[31]. The chemical nature of the substances involved has recently been elucidated, and two forms of inhibin have been identified. The overall present evidence suggests that inhibin is important in the regulation of FSH responses to GnRH, although the exact role of inhibin *in vivo* is presently uncertain.

CONCLUSIONS

The regulation of the normal menstrual cycle consists of a complex series of interactions between the hypothalamus, pituitary and ovaries, and changes in the pattern of GnRH secretion appear to play an important role in the ability of GnRH to modify the number of its own receptors. In addition, steroid modulation of receptor numbers and sensitivity all account for the complex changes seen in LH and FSH levels throughout the menstrual cycle. Many factors can alter this complex and sensitive control of the hypothalamic–pituitary axis with resultant disorders in GnRH secretion or altered sensitivity of the pituitary gonadotrophs. Conditions with abnormal levels of ovarian steroids, adrenal or thyroid hormones can all result in disruption of normal gonadotrophin stimulation of follicular growth and maturation and many common disorders seen in clinical practice will be discussed in subsequent chapters of this book.

REFERENCES

1. Midgley, A.R. and Jaffe, R.B. (1971). Regulation of human gonadotrophins – episodic fluctuation of LH during the menstrual cycle. *J. Clin. Endocrinol. Metab.*, **33**, 962–9
2. Clarke, I.J. and Cummins, J.T. (1982). The temporal relationship between gonadotrophin releasing hormone (GnRH) and luteinizing hormone (LH) secretion in ovariectomized ewes. *Endocrinology*, **111**, 1737–9
3. Belchetz, P.E., Plant, T.M., Nakai, Y., Keogh, E.G. and Knobil, E. (1978). Hypophysical responses to continuous and intermittent delivery of hypothalamic gonadotrophin-releasing hormone. *Science*, **202**, 631–3
4. Leyendecker, G., Wildt, L. and Hansmen, M. (1980). Pregnancies following intermittent pulsatile administration of GnRH. *J. Clin. Endocrinol. Metab.*, **51**, 1214–16

5. Wildt, L., Hausler, A., Marshall, G., Hutchinson, J.S., Plant, T.M., Belchetz, P.E. and Knobil, E. (1981). Frequency and amplitude of gonadotrophin releasing hormone stimulation and gonadotrophin secretion in the rhesus monkey. *Endocrinology*, **109**, 376–85

6. Grossman, A., Moult, P.J.A., Gaillard, R.C., Delitala, G., Toff, W.D., Rees, L.H. and Besser, G.M. (1981). The opioid control of LH and FSH release – effects of a met-enkephalin analogue and naloxone. *Clin. Endocrinol.*, **14**, 41–7

7. Neill, J.D., Patton, J.M., Daily, R.A., Tsou, R.C. and Tindall, G.T. (1977). Luteinizing hormone-releasing hormone (LHRH) in pituitary stalk blood of rhesus monkeys – relationship to level of LH release. *Endocrinology*, **101**, 430–4

8. Sarker, D.K., Chiappa, S.A., Fink, G. and Shrewood, N.M. (1975). Gonadotrophin releasing hormone surge in proestrous rats. *Nature (London)*, **264**, 461–3

9. Backstrom, C.T., McNeilly, A.S., Leask, R.M. and Baird, D.T. (1982). Pulsatile secretion of LH, FSH, prolactin, estradiol and progesterone during the human menstrual cycle. *Clin. Endocrinol.*, **17**, 29–38

10. Karsch, F.J., Foster, D.K., Bittman, E.L. and Goodman, R.L. (1983). A role for estradiol in enhancing luteinizing hormone pulse frequency during the follicular phase of the estrous cycle of sheep. *Endocrinology*, **113**, 1333–9

11. Goodman, R.L. and Karsch, F.J. (1980). Pulsatile secretion of luteinizing hormone – differential suppression by ovarian steroids. *Endocrinology*, **107**, 1286–92

12. Soules, M.R., Steiner, R.A., Clifton, D.K., Cohen, N.L., Anksel, S. and Bremner, W.J. (1984). Progesterone modulation of pulsatile luteinizing secretion in normal women. *J. Clin. Endocrinol. Metab.*, **58**, 378–83

13. Odell, W.D. and Swerdloff, R.S. (1968). Progesterone-induced luteinizing and follicle-stimulating hormone surge in post-menopausal women – a stimulated ovulatory peak. *Proc. Natl. Acad. Sci. USA*, **61**, 529–36

14. Sauder, S.E., Frager, M., Case, G.D., Kelch, R.P. and Marshall, J.C. (1984). Abnormal patterns of pulsatile luteinizing hormone secretion in women with hyperprolactinemia and amenorrhoea – responses to bromocriptine. *J. Clin. Endocrinol. Metab.*, **59**, 941–8

15. Marian, J. and Conn, P.M. (1983). Subcellular localisation of the receptor for gonadotrophin-releasing hormone in pituitary and ovarian tissue. *Endocrinology*, **112**, 104–12

16. Eidne, K.A., Sellar, R.E., Couper, G., Anderson, L. and Taylor, P.L. (1992). Molecular cloning and characterisation of the rat pituitary gonadotrophin-releasing hormone (GnRH) receptor. *Mol. Cell. Endocrinol.*, **90**, R5–R9

17. Clayton, R.N., Detta, A., Naik, S.I., Young, S. and Charlton, H.M. (1985). Gonadotrophin–releasing hormone receptor regulation and relationship to gonadotrophin secretion. *J. Steroid Biochem.*, **23**, 691–702

18. Young, L.S., Speight, A., Charlton, H.M. and Clayton, R.N. (1983). Pituitary gonadotrophin–releasing hormone receptor regulation in the hypogonadotrophic hypergonadal (hpg) mouse. *Endocrinology*, **113**, 55–61

19. Clayton, R.N., Solano, A.R., Garcia-Vela, A., Dufau, M. and Catt, K.J. (1980). Regulation of pituitary receptors for gonadotrophin–releasing hormone during the rat estrous cycle. *Endocrinology*, **107**, 699–706

20. Adams, T.E., Norman, R.L. and Spies, H.G. (1981). Gonadotrophin–releasing hormone receptor binding and pituitary responsiveness in estrodiol-primed monkeys. *Science*, **213**, 1388–90

21. Clayton, R.N. (1982). Gonadotrophin–releasing hormone modulation of its own pituitary receptors: evidence for biphasic regulation. *Endocrinology*, **111**, 152–61

22. Gorospe, W.C. and Conn, M. (1987). Agents that decrease gonadotrophin–releasing hormone (GnRH) receptor internalization do not inhibit GnRH-medicated gonadotrope desensitisation. *Endocrinology*, **120**, 222–9

23. Chang, J.P., McCoy, E.E., Graeter, J., Tasaka, K. and Catt, K.J. (1986). Participation of voltage-dependent calcium channels in the action of gonadotrophin releasing hormone. *J. Biol. Chem.*, **261**, 9105–8

24. Berridge, M.J. (1984). Inositol triphosphate and diacylglycerol as second messengers. *Biochem. J.*, **220**, 345–60

25. Abbot, S.D., Doherty, K., Roberts, J.L., Tepper, M.A., Chin, W.W. and Clayton, R.N. (1985). Castration increases luteinizing hormone subunit messenger RNA levels in male rat pituitaries. *J. Endocrinol.*, **107**, R1–R4

26. Ramey, J.W., Highsmith, R.F., Wilfinger, W.W. and Baldwin, D.M. (1987). The effects of gonadotrophin–releasing hormone and estradiol on luteinizing biosynthesis in cultured rat anterior pituitary cells. *Endocrinology*, **120**, 1503–13

27. Shaw, R.W., Butt, W.R., London, D.R. and Marshall, J.C. (1974). Variation in response to synthetic luteinizing hormone-releasing hormone (LH-RH) at different phases of the same menstrual cycle in normal women. *J. Obstet. Gynaecol. Br. Commwlth.*, **81**, 632–9

28. Shaw, R.W., Butt, W.R. and London, D.R. (1975). The effect of estrogen pretreatment on subsequent response to luteinizing hormone-releasing hormone in normal women. *Clin. Endocrinol.*, **4**, 297–304

29. Shaw, R.W., Butt, W.R. and London, D.R. (1975). Effect of progesterone on FSH and LH response to LH-RH in normal women. *Clin. Endocrinol.*, **4**, 543–50

30. Duncan, J.A., Barkan, A., Herbon, L. and Marshall, J.C. (1986). Regulation of pituitary GnRH receptors by pulsatile GnRH in female rats: effects of estradiol and prolactin. *Endocrinology*, **118**, 320–7

31. Hoffman, J.C., Lorenzen, J.R., Weil, T. and Schwartz, N.B. (1979). Selective suppression of the primary surge of follicle-stimulating hormone in the rat – further evidence for folliculostatin in porcine follicular fluid. *Endocrinology*, **105**, 200–3

32. Clayton, R.N. (1989). Cellular actions of gonadotrophin-releasing hormone: the receptor and beyond. In Shaw, R.W. and Marshall, J.C. (eds.) *LHRH and its Analogues*, p. 29. (London: Wright/Butterworths)

33. Clarke, I.J. and Cummins, J.T. (1984). Direct pituitary effects of estrogen and progesterone on gonadotropin secretion in the ovariectomized ewe. *Neuroendocrinology*, **39**, 267–74

2

Congenital pituitary endocrine failure

P.-M.G. Bouloux, V. Duke and R. Quinton

INTRODUCTION

Congenital pituitary failure can result from primary hypothalamic deficiency of one or more pituitary releasing hormones or factors, or from a specific pituitary defect leading to deficiency of hypophyseal hormone release. Although congenital deficiency of growth hormone (GH) and adrenocorticotrophic hormone (ACTH) secretion have been reported, hypogonadism due to deficiency of luteinizing hormone (LH) and follicle stimulating hormone (FSH) constitutes one of the most frequent forms of congenital pituitary failure, and leads to hypogonadotrophic hypogonadism. As in the case of GH and ACTH deficiency, the defect resides in the hypothalamus, with failed synthesis and/or release of hypothalamo-hypophysiotropic hormones. This can be inferred from the observation that exogenous administration of growth hormone releasing hormone (GHRH), corticotrophin releasing hormone (CRH) and gonadotrophin releasing hormone (GnRH) can stimulate release of their respective pituitary hormones in such cases. Theoretically, mutations within or deletions of the gene for pituitary receptors for hypothalamic releasing hormones could be responsible for pituitary failure but, hitherto, none has been described.

17

GnRH DEFICIENCY

GnRH deficiency can occur sporadically or in an inherited manner. In the latter case, familial studies suggest a predominantly X-linked mode of transmission, and molecular genetic studies have implicated a locus distal to the Duchenne muscular dystrophy gene as being causal. Kallmann's syndrome, or olfactogenital dysplasia, is a genetic disorder of neuronal migration in which, during embryogenesis, GnRH cells fail to migrate from the medial olfactory placode along the terminalis and vomeronasal nerves into the septopreoptic area of the anterior hypothalamus. Further, projections from the lateral olfactory placode fail to induce the development of the olfactory bulbs. Phenotypically, affected patients have hypogonadotrophic hypogonadism in association with anosmia/hyposmia. The simultaneous occurrence of absent olfactory bulbs and tracts with sexual infantilism was first documented in a male autopsy in 1856[1]. In 1944, the heritable nature of this condition was first elucidated[2]. The hypogonadism of Kallmann's syndrome thus results from lack of secretion of the hypothalamo-hypophysiotrophic hormone GnRH, causing inappropriately low gonadotrophin levels and absence of any discernible pulsatility of LH and FSH. Patients rarely present with olfactory disturbance as a symptom, and more usually the diagnosis is established during investigation of hypogonadism (in the male, micropenis, cryptorchidism, delayed puberty, arrested puberty or infertility). That deficient GnRH secretion underpins hypogonadism is suggested by the ability of low-dose pulsatile GnRH therapy to reverse the hypogonadotrophic state in both sexes and induce sexual maturation[3,4]. Although isolated hypogonadotrophic hypogonadism with anosmia/hyposmia is recognized in the female, where it usually presents with delayed puberty and primary amenorrhoea, it is considerably more rare, and is not discussed in this review, which specifically focuses on Kallmann's syndrome affecting the male.

Classification

Kallmann's syndrome is relatively uncommon, occurring in 1 in 10 000 males and 1 in 50 000 females[5,6]. The condition usually occurs sporadically, but may be inherited, usually as an X-linked trait (XKS);

autosomal recessive and dominant modes of inheritance have also been described[7-9]. The approximately 5–7-fold excess in male preponderance supports the contention that the X-linked form of the condition predominates. In our experience, out of 58 fully ascertained cases, nine individuals gave a family history indicative of an X-linked recessive disorder, with an autosomal dominant mode of inheritance discernible in only one pedigree. The remaining cases were sporadic. We have also seen one set of identical twins *discordant* for the Kallmann's syndrome phenotype.

Contiguous gene abnormalities and Kallmann's syndrome

In the majority of familial cases, Kallmann's syndrome occurs as an isolated abnormality. However, several pedigrees have been documented where hypogonadotrophic hypogonadism occurred in conjunction with one or more phenotypic abnormalities, including congenital ichthyosis (due to steroid sulphatase deficiency), mild mental retardation, chondrodysplasia punctata, and hypopigmentation of the iris[10-12]. The genetic basis of these co-inherited abnormalities usually resides in a microdeletion in the Xp22.3 region, often with loss of several megabases of DNA containing contiguous genes. The pedigree described by Sunohara and colleagues[11] was notable for the co-inheritance of ichthyosis, anosmia, nystagmus with decreased visual acuity, strabismus, hypopigmentation of the iris, and mirror movements of the hands and *feet*. This association suggests a more extensive genetic lesion than hitherto described; no molecular genetic studies have been reported in this pedigree, however. Deletion analysis of patients with these contiguous gene syndromes has played a key role enabling assignment of the order of loci in the Xp22.3 region, and the identification of the minimum interval of DNA incorporating the Kallmann gene[13,14]. An additional important clinical point, however, is that the obligate heterozygote mothers of males with contiguous gene abnormalities and steroid sulphatase deficiency I (causing ichthyosis) are susceptible to prolonged labour, due to cervical dystocia. The obstetrician thus needs to be alerted to the increased foetal risks in such mothers.

Clinical manifestations of X-linked Kallmann's syndrome

We have studied 58 patients with isolated Kallmann's syndrome, and two families in whom Kallmann's syndrome was inherited as part of a contiguous gene abnormality. Nine pedigrees with an X-linked mode of inheritance were detected and their phenotype is discussed below. Abnormalities referable to the central nervous and urogenital systems were consistently found and are in agreement with previous reports[9,15]. These associated defects were most consistent in cases of XKS, in which discordance of these associated phenotypes could be observed even within affected members of the same pedigree.

Neurological manifestations

Olfactory function in patients and carriers

We have tested olfaction using seven odorants at six concentrations[16] in patients, their unaffected sibs and parents. We have noted complete anosmia to all concentrations of the seven different odorants in all affected cases, but in XKS, subnormal sensitivity of smell in the female obligate heterozygotes was documented when compared with normal controls[17]. Given that the obligate carriers appear to have intact olfactory tracts and bulbs, the interpretation of these findings is at present unclear.

Olfactory mucosa

A recent study by Schwob and colleagues[18] has reported on the histopathological appearance of the olfactory mucosa in a single case of Kallmann's syndrome in which absence of olfactory bulbs had been confirmed on magnetic resonance imaging (MRI) scanning. Biopsy of the olfactory mucosa revealed defective olfactory neurones. Most of these lacked cilia (i.e. were morphologically immature). The fila olfactoria had fewer than the normal number of axons and a large number were apparently undergoing electron-lucent degeneration. Finally, neuromatous collections were seen superficial to the basement membrane of the epithelium. Similar changes have been observed in the mucosa of

Table 1 Neurological abnormalities in Kallmann's syndrome

Hereditary bimanual synkinesis
Visuospatial abnormalities
Saccadic dysmetria
Gaze-invoked horizontal nystagmus
Impaired smooth pursuit
Sensorineural hearing loss
Seizures
Suprasellar Rathke's pouch cysts
Right cerebral hemiatrophy
Retinitis pigmentosa
Pes cavus deformity of the feet

experimentally bulbectomized rodents. It thus appears that the changes observed in Kallmann's syndrome are characteristic of olfactory mucosa that cannot innervate the olfactory bulb in both humans and animals. The appearances of olfactory mucosa in this study were very similar to those seen in a 19-week-old affected foetus[19].

Other neurological defects

Detailed neurological examinations and MRI of the brain were performed in several of our patients with isolated XKS and those with contiguous gene abnormalities. Abnormalities recorded by ourselves and others[15] are listed in Table 1. Synkinesis was assessed by asking subjects to perform unilateral intentional movements. Typically, this included finger tapping, rapid trigger movements of the forefinger, repetitive flexion–extension of the wrists, supination–pronation of the forearm, and flexion–extension at the elbow. Unilateral movements of each foot, including wiggling of the toes, and flexion–extension and eversion–inversion of the ankles were also performed. Synkinesis was considered present if any of the corresponding muscles of the contralateral extremity moved in unison with the primary movement. Hereditary bimanual synkinesis was observed in only XKS with a penetrance of 74% and was not seen in sporadic cases; it thus appears to be a specific marker for XKS.

The severity of synkinesis within pedigrees was noted to be variable, some individuals being only very mildly affected, others finding this symptom disabling. It is of interest that some patients are unaware of mirror movements, although their parents often note difficulty with such activities as piano playing and front-crawl swimming.

Neurological basis of synkinesis

The precise anatomical areas responsible for mirror movements are not as yet identified. One theory[20] suggests that they arise from a lack of inhibitory fibres within the corpus callosum. These fibres are thought to originate in one hemisphere, pass through the corpus callosum and inhibit the contralateral uncrossed pyramidal tract. It is of interest that mirror movements have been described in patients with agenesis of the corpus callosum, and they are commonly present in young children but disappear at approximately 10 years of age, when myelination of the corpus callosum is complete. Shibakasu and Nahgae[20] have investigated movement-related potentials in an affected patient. In normal subjects, a pre-movement negative wave, corresponding to preparatory excitation of the motor cortex, was observed in only the hemisphere contralateral to the side of intended movement. In the patient with Kallmann's syndrome, this pre-movement potential was recorded bilaterally, signifying synchronous excitation of both frontal motor strips. MRI scans performed in 10 patients with both sporadic and X-linked Kallmann's syndrome have failed to demonstrate the absence, or consistent morphological abnormalities, of the corpus callosum (Bouloux and Matfin, unpublished observations) to support this hypothesis. An alternative explanation for synkinesis suggests an underlying inadequate pyramidal decussation[21]. While there are suggestions that this mechanism may be responsible for mirror movements in the Klippel–Feil syndrome, there are no published morphological, neurophysiological or neuro-radiological data to support this hypothesis in Kallmann's syndrome.

Magnetic resonance abnormalities

The only abnormalities noted on MRI scans of our patients have been occasional thinning of the corpus callosum, and uniform absence of

Table 2 Morphological and histological abnormalities of testes in Kallmann's syndrome

Reduced/absent Leydig cells
Decreased seminiferous tubule numbers
Decreased spermatocyte formation
Peritubular fibrosis and hyalinization
Absent vas deferens
Absent testes

olfactory sulci. Axial T_1-weighted images through the expected location of the olfactory bulbs and tracts showed only subarachnoid fluid lateral to the crista galli. In a recent series of nine cases[22] using a 1.5-T magnet, dysplastic tangles in the region of the cribriform plate were also observed in 30% of cases. These may correspond to the neuromatous tangles observed by Schwanzel-Fukuda[23] in an affected 19-week male foetus.

Urogenital abnormalities

Unilateral renal agenesis occurring in X-linked or male-sex-limited dominant euneuchoidal hypogonadism was first noted by Sainton[24] in 1902. Its occurrence in a fully ascertained case of Kallmann's syndrome was first noted by Nowakowski and Lenz[25] and in familial Kallmann's syndrome by Wegenke and associates[26], who documented a pedigree in which two brothers and their double first cousin had Kallmann's syndrome and unilateral renal agenesis, associated in one with unilateral absence of a testis. The testicular biopsy in one untreated affected male (performed during orchidopexy at age 11), showed a conspicuous absence of Leydig cells, decreased numbers of seminiferous tubules, and marked decrease of spermatocyte formation. Abnormalities of testicular morphology and histology previously documented in Kallmann's syndrome are shown in Table 2. We have investigated several of our patients for renal agenesis using ultrasonography or dimenaptosuccinic acid (DMSA) scanning. The abnormality was only found in patients with XKS as an isolated abnormality, or as part of a contiguous gene abnormality. In our pedigrees, a striking feature has been the approximately

Table 3   Abnormalities reported in Kallmann's syndrome

Hypogonadotrophic hypogonadism
Anosmia
Cryptorchidism
Urological abnormalities
CNS abnormalities
Choanal atresia
Cleft lip and palate
Malrotation of the gut

50% penetrance of renal agenesis, even within pedigrees. This occurred irrespective of whether the underlying genetic defect was a microdeletion of the entire gene, or whether a point mutation was involved. This strongly suggests that absence of the gene can be compensated for in some individuals, and raises the possible involvement of epigenetic phenomena in renal development.

Other associations

Kallmann's syndrome has been described in association with a number of other phenotypic abnormalities (Table 3). These include choanal atresia, cleft lip and palate, malrotation of the gut and shortened fourth metacarpals. However, since these associations are rare, it seems unlikely that they form part of the syndrome proper.

Hypogonadism and its management

Kallmann's syndrome presents clinically in a variety of ways, and at different ages. In the male, micropenis, undescended testes (cryptorchidism), delayed puberty, arrested puberty, and infertility comprise the clinical manifestations of the associated hypogonadism. In the adolescent or young adult male, treatment objectives are, first, to restore normal serum androgen levels, allowing virilization and puberty to be accomplished, and, second, to induce fertility where appropriate. Treatment for cryptorchidism should ideally have been undertaken early on.

Table 4   Treatment modalities for hypogonadism in Kallmann's syndrome

Testosterone
Human chorionic gonadotrophins
GnRH therapy
    s.c., thrice daily
    pulsatile s.c. or i.v.
    intranasal
hCG + hMG i.m. or s.c.

Treatment modalities

These are listed in Table 4.

Pulsatile GnRH therapy

The deficiency of a normal pulsatile delivery of GnRH from the portal circulation to the pituitary in both idiopathic hypogonadotrophic hypogonadism (IHH) and Kallmann's syndrome has proved a logical starting point for the use of exogenous pulsatile GnRH therapy in the induction of pubertal development and acquisition of fertility in affected patients of both sexes. Based on normative data, the frequency of subcutaneous (s.c.) or intravenous (i.v.) GnRH administration demonstrated to be effective in men with GnRH deficiency was 2-hourly. Increases or decreases in this frequency resulted in deviations from normal of both gonadotrophin and testosterone levels. Treatment has been given both i.v. and s.c. in various studies.

Pulsatile GnRH therapy using variable boluses ranging from 25–600 ng/kg/bolus has been reported to yield a 100% response in stimulating pituitary output of gonadotrophins and testicular steroid production in a group of 51 unselected patients with IHH[3]. Factors correlating with the magnitude of the effective individual GnRH doses included body weight (positively) and initial testicular volume (negatively). Patients with the largest initial gonadal size had the most rapid rate of testicular growth, although individual patients with smaller initial testicular volumes could also achieve normal gonadal size. Spermatogenesis induction was successful in this series in 34/51 patients; of the remainder, two had severe cryptorchidism without significant testicular growth, three remained azoospermic after 8–18 months' treatment, and six had been on treatment for less than 6 months. The time between initiation of GnRH therapy and the appearance of sperm in the ejaculate ranged from 18–139 weeks, depending largely on the size of the pre-therapy gonad. The authors state that it was uncommon to see sperm production in testes less than 8 ml. An important clinical point emerging from these studies was that excellent fertility potential could be achieved despite low sperm counts.

GnRH versus gonadotrophin therapy

A comparison of GnRH therapy with gonadotrophin therapy has been reported in males with IHH[27]. Eighteen patients of matched age and similar testicular volume were treated in each group. Pulsatile GnRH therapy was initiated with 4 µg GnRH s.c. every 2 h and gonadotrophin therapy with 3×2500 IU human chorionic gonadotrophin (hCG) weekly, injected intramuscularly (i.m.). After 8–12 weeks of hCG therapy, 150 IU human menopausal gonadotrophins (hMG) were injected 2–4 times weekly. Testosterone (T) and estradiol (E_2) levels were significantly higher (T: $p < 0.03$; E_2: $p < 0.001$) in the gonadotrophin group than in the pulsatile GnRH group (T: 22.5 ± 8.1 versus 16.8 ± 5.5 nmol/l; E_2: 150 ± 70 versus 88 ± 59 pmol/l). Five patients developed gynaecomastia during gonadotrophin therapy. The rise in testicular volume was significantly more pronounced in the GnRH group (Δ testicular volume 8.1 ± 2.0 ml) than in the gonadotrophin group (Δ testicular volume $= 4.8 \pm 1.8$ ml). Ten of the GnRH and eight of the gonadotrophin group had positive sperm counts, of $1.5–26 \times 10^6$/ml. Positive sperm counts were achieved more rapidly in the GnRH group (12 ± 1.6 versus 20 ± 2.3 months; $p < 0.02$). In another 2-year comparative study, using smaller groups of patients, Liu and colleagues[28] found the opposite effect, with gonadotrophin therapy resulting in a superior response in terms of testicular growth and degree of spermatogenesis. One problem with interpretation of studies using either GnRH or gonadotrophin therapy has been the absence of standardization of the doses used and, indeed, duration of treatment. Other confounding factors affecting the outcome of treatment are shown in Table 5. Some regimens have used as little as 1 ampoule of hMG three times a week, others 4 ampoules three times weekly. Furthermore, few studies have

Table 5 Confounding factors in the interpretation of the results of therapy in males with idiopathic hypogonadotrophic hypogonadism

Lack of homogeneity of patient groups
    previous orchidopexy
    previous therapy
    initial testicular volume
Small numbers treated
Variation in treatment regimes
Variation in treatment duration

attempted to address the therapeutic response specifically in patients with Kallmann's syndrome, who have a higher incidence of cryptorchidism than patients with IHH.

Cryptorchidism

In our experience, the incidence of unilateral or bilateral cryptorchidism is 56% in sporadic Kallmann's syndrome and reaches 85% in XKS, compared with an incidence of 15% in IHH. There is ample evidence that the spermatogenetic response to physiological (endogenous) and exogenous stimulant therapy is poor in this patient group[29]. Abnormal hypothalamic–pituitary testicular function has been demonstrated within the first year of life in many children with cryptorchidism. Gendrel and associates[30] have documented plasma gonadotrophin and testosterone levels from day 30–120 in 57 term male infants born with undescended testes (bilateral in 22 and unilateral in 35). Clinical follow-up of these infants showed that spontaneous testicular descent occurred in 27 at 2–4 months; the 30 others remained cryptorchid at 6 months. Plasma LH and the postnatal rise in testosterone were significantly lower in patients remaining cryptorchid, either unilaterally or bilaterally, than in infants with delayed spontaneous descent of one or both testes. These data suggest a primary LH deficiency in cryptorchidism, a defect that is likely to be even more accentuated in Kallmann's syndrome.

It is well established that fertility is impaired in the cryptorchid male[29]. Contemporary reviews have shown that 50% of males with unilateral cryptorchidism, and 75% of males with bilateral cryptorchidism suffer from fertility impairment. It is notable that progressive histological deterioration of the cryptorchid testes occurs within the first year of life. The mean number of germ cells in cryptorchid and normal testes remain approximately the same for the first 6 months of life, but differences exist by the 12th month. By the age of 2, marked germinal atrophy is already present in 40%. Progressive, continued loss of germ cells occurs during childhood so that the adult cryptorchid testes are uniformly devoid of cells. Leydig cell atrophy is also a prominent feature.

Induction of fertility with gonadotrophins

We have recently reported on a series of 26 male patients with IHH, aged 17–48 years at assessment[17]. Patients were divided according to whether they had cryptorchidism (group 1) or not (group 2). In group 1, seven had unilateral and six had bilateral cryptorchidism. Of these patients, 11/13 satisfied the diagnostic criteria for Kallmann's syndrome. This had been treated at presentation with orchidopexy in eight and with hCG injections in two. Ten patients in this group had previously received therapy with testosterone and, in addition, four had also received therapy with hCG, and two with s.c. GnRH. Only one patient in group 2 was hyposmic. All patients, in both groups, in whom seminal analyses were performed were azoospermic. Although some of these patients had been treated with testosterone previously, it is known that prior androgen exposure does not impair subsequent spermatogenesis[31].

Following clinical and endocrine assessment, 11 patients in group 1 and 12 in group 2 were treated using a standard protocol of hCG 2000 IU i.m., twice-weekly for 6 weeks, followed by 1000 IU twice-weekly. Four patients in group 1 and five patients in group 2 requested treatment to promote fertility and received therapy with combined hCG (500 IU twice weekly) and hMG (Pergonal® 4 ampoules thrice-weekly). There was no significant difference between groups 1 and 2 in basal levels of LH, FSH, or peak levels of gonadotrophin (both of which were subnormal in both groups) after 100 µg i.v. GnRH. In the hCG-stimulation tests, the testosterone response was greater in group 2 than group 1, but this did not reach statistical significance.

Patients in group 2 responded to hCG therapy with a greater increase in testicular volume than in group 1 (4.7 ± 1.8 versus 3.0 ± 1.6 ml:

$p < 0.02$). Interestingly, there was no difference in the response of patients who had had unilateral or bilateral cryptorchidism, or between those who had previously had surgery or hCG therapy. During hCG therapy, the maximum serum testosterone level rose into the normal range in only three out of 13 patients in group 1 compared with six patients in group 2.

With respect to the spermatogenetic response to combined hCG and hMG therapy, only 6/9 patients achieved spermatogenesis; 1/4 in group 1 and 5/5 in group 2. All patients in group 2 achieved significant spermatogenesis with 10–14 months of hCG/hMG therapy. The partners of three of them became pregnant. The remaining two achieved spermatogenesis but had sperm counts of less than 1×10^6/ml. These observations emphasize the poor outcome of spermatogenesis induction in Kallmann's syndrome. However, it is unclear whether previous cryptorchidism (and indeed its surgical management) was solely responsible, or whether the severe nature of the gonadotrophin deficiency characteristic of Kallmann's syndrome also played a role.

There is now evidence that the neonatal surge of LH and testosterone may play an important role in priming the subsequent Leydig/Sertoli/germ cell function in puberty. In the rhesus monkey, suppression of the neonatal LH/testosterone surge by pituitary downregulation with a superactive GnRH analogue has been shown to impair subsequent spermatogenesis during sexual maturation[32]. It is tempting to speculate that the pubertal spermatogenic response to stimulant therapy might be enhanced in patients with Kallmann's syndrome with early treatment of cryptorchidism, and the use of hCG to stimulate and mimic the physiological surge of testosterone in the first few months of life. However, this would depend on being able to diagnose the condition accurately early in life, and although such attempts have been reported[33] this remains a difficult clinical area.

PRESENT AND FUTURE CONSIDERATIONS

Recent data, presented in this chapter, suggest that the X-linked form of Kallmann's syndrome results from defective expression of a protein with cell adhesion-like properties[13,14]. Molecular genetic studies carried out in collaboration with Petit's group in the Pasteur Institute in Paris have resulted in the identification of several individuals with deletions of the

Xp22.3 region and point mutations of the Kalig 1 gene in others. There is, however, no hot spot for mutations among the 14 exons of the XKS gene. The pioneering work of Schwanzel-Fukuda and Pfaff[23] has demonstrated that GnRH cells have their origin in the medial olfactory placode of the olfactory pit, and subsequently migrate along the nervus terminalis and vomeronasal nerves to the septopreoptic region of the hypothalamus. The finding of arrested migration of GnRH cells at the cribriform plate in a 19-week-old Kallmann foetus led to the hypothesis that failure of a putative adhesion molecule might underpin this GnRH migration defect in Kallmann's syndrome, as well as leading to defective induction of the olfactory bulb and tract during development. The cloning of the X-linked Kallmann gene, together with the homology of the encoded protein with cell adhesion molecules, has substantiated this hypothesis.

It would appear, however, that the X-linked Kallmann gene is involved in the development of other important biological functions. Hereditary bimanual synkinesis (mirror movements) may have its origins in the failure of axonal guidance and migration, and the Kallmann protein thus appears to have a role in the organization and functioning of the pyramidal pathways. The role of the Kallmann protein in renal development is more obscure. The Kallmann gene transcript has been detected in the kidney, but its absence can be totally compensated for. Further studies are required to investigate its expression and role in the developing kidney. The high incidence of cryptorchidism has not been fully explained. Whether it relates to the severe gonadotrophin (and thus testosterone) deficiency *in utero*, or failure of the gubernacular development (possibly cell adhesion mediated) remains to be elucidated. In general, the poor response of this group of patients to spermatogenesis induction suggests that alternative earlier and more aggressive therapeutic approaches (see above) should be considered. However, such options depend upon the ability to make an early diagnosis. It seems likely that future progress in molecular genetics – specifically the identification of additional loci responsible for Kallmann's syndrome – will critically improve our ability to achieve this goal.

ACKNOWLEDGEMENTS

We are grateful to Professor Michael Besser, Dr Martin Savage, Dr Steve Shalet, Dr Owen Edwards, and Professor Howard Jacobs for allowing us to report on their patients.

REFERENCES

1. Maestre San Juan, A. (1856). Teratologia: falta total de los nervios olfactorios con anosmia ennun individuo en quien existia un atrofia congenita de los testiculos y miembro viril. *Siglo Med.*, **3**, 211

2. Kallmann, F.J., Schoenfeld, W.A. and Barrere, S.E. (1944). The genetic aspects of primary euneuchoidism. *Am. J. Ment. Defic.*, **48**, 203–6

3. Hoffmann, A.R. and Crowley, W.F. (1982). Induction of puberty in men by long term pulsatile administration of low-dose gonadotrophin releasing hormone. *N. Engl. J. Med.*, **307**, 1237–41

4. Spratt, D., Finkelstein, J.S., O'Dea, L.S.L, Badger, T.M., Rao, P.N., Campbell, J.D. and Crowley, W.F. (1986). Long term administration of gonadotrophin releasing hormone in men with idiopathic hypogonado-trophic hypogonadism. *Ann. Intern. Med.*, **105**, 848–52

5. Jones, J.R. and Kemmann, E. (1976). Olfactogenital dysplasia in the female. *Obstet. Gynaecol. Ann.*, **5**, 443–6

6. Pawlowitzki, I.H., Diekstall, P., Schadel, A. and Miny, P. (1987). Estimating the frequency of Kallmann syndrome among hypogonadal and among anosmic patients. *Am. J. Hum. Genet.*, **26**, 473–9

7. Sparkes, R.S., Simpson, R.W. and Paulsen, C.A. (1968). Familial hypo-gonadotrophic hypogonadism with anosmia. *Arch. Intern. Med.*, **21**, 534–8

8. Santen, R.J. and Paulsen, C.A. (1973). Hypogonadotrophic hypogonadism 1. Clinical study of the mode of inheritance. *J. Clin. Endocrinol. Metab.*, **36**, 47–52

9. White, B.J., Rogol, A.D., Brown, K.S., Lieblich, J.M. and Rosen, S. (1983). The syndrome of anosmia and hypogonadotrophic hypogonadism: a genetic study of 18 new families and a review. *Am. J. Med. Genet.*, **15**, 417–35

10. Rud, E. (1927). Tilfaelde af Infantilisme med Tetani, Epilepsi, Polyneurtis, ichthyosis og anaemi af pernicious Type. *Hospitalstidende*, **70**, 525–38

11. Sunohara, N., Sakuragawa, N., Satayoshi, E., Tanae, A. and Shapiro, L.J. (1986). A new syndrome of anosmia, ichthyosis, hypogonadism and various neurological manifestations with deficiency of steroid sulfatase and aryl sulphatase C. *Ann. Neurol.*, **19**, 174–81

12. Bouloux, P.-M.G., Kirk, J.M.W., Munroe, P., Duke, V., Meindl, A., Hilson, A., Grant, D., Carter, N., Betts, D., Meitinger, T. and Besser, G.M. (1993). Deletion analysis maps ocular albinism proximal to the steroid sulphatase locus. *Clin. Genet.*, **43**, 169–74

13. Legouis, R., Hardelin, J.P., Levilliers, J., Claverie, J.-M., Compain, S., Wunderle, V., Milasseau, P., Le Paslier, D., Cohen, D., Bouguerelet, L., Delamare-van der Waal, H., Lutlalla, G., Weissenbach, J. and Petit, C.

(1991). The candidate gene for the X-linked Kallmann's syndrome encodes a protein related to adhesion molecules. *Cell*, **67**, 423–35

14. Franco, B., Guioli, S., Pragliola, A., Incerti, B., Bardoni, B., Tonlorenzi, R., Carrozzo, R., Maestrini, E., Pieretti, M., Taillon Miller, P., Brown, C.J., Willard, H.F., Lawrence, C., Persico, M.G., Camerino, G. and Ballabio, A. (1991). A gene deleted in Kallmann's syndrome shares homology with neural cell adhesion and axonal path binding molecules. *Nature (London)*, **353**, 529–36

15. Schwankhaus, J.D., Currie, J., Jaffe, M.J., Rose, S.R. and Sherins, R.J. (1989). Neurological findings in men with isolated hypogonadotrophic hypogonadism. *Neurology*, **39**, 223–9

16. Rosen, S.W., Gann, P. and Rogol, A.D. (1979). Congenital anosmia: detection threshold for seven odorant classes in hypogonadal and eugonadal patients. *Ann. Otol.*, **88**, 288–92

17. Kirk, J.M.W., Grant, D.B., Savage, M.D., Besser, G.M. and Bouloux, G.-M. (1993). Olfactory dysfunction in carriers of X-linked Kallmann's syndrome. *Clin. Endocrinol.*, in press

18. Schwob, J.E., Leopold, D.A., Szumowski, K.E.M. and Emko, P. (1994). Histopathology of olfactory mucosa in Kallmann's Syndrome. *Ann. Otorhinolaryngol.*, **102**, 117–22

19. Schwanzel-Fukuda, M., Bick, D. and Pfaff, D.W. (1989). Luteinizing hormone releasing hormone (LNRH)-expressing cells do not migrate normally in an inherited hypogonadal (Kallmann) syndrome. *Molec. Brain Res.*, **6**, 311–25

20. Shibakasu, H. and Nahgae, K. (1984). Mirror movement: application of movement-related cortical potentials. *Ann. Neurol.*, **15**, 299–302

21. Conrad, B., Kriebel, J. and Hetzel, W.D. (1978). Hereditary bimanual synkineses combined with hypogonadotrophic hypogonadism and anosmia in four brothers. *J. Neurol.*, **218**, 263–74

22. Truwit, C.L., Barkowich, A.J., Grumbach, M.M. and Martini, J.J. (1993). MR imaging of Kallmann syndrome, a genetic disorder of neuronal migration affecting the olfactory and genital systems. *Am. J. Neuroradiol.*, **14**, 827–38

23. Schwanzel-Fukuda, M. and Pfaff, D.W. (1989). Origin of luteinizing hormone releasing hormone. *Nature (London)*, **338**, 161–4

24. Sainton, P. (1902). Un cas d'euneuchisme familial. *Nouv. Iconogr. Salpet.*, **15**, 272–7

25. Nowakowski, H. and Lenz, W. (1961). Genetic aspects in male hypogonadism. *Rec. Prog. Horm. Res.*, **17**, 53–95

26. Wegenke, J.D., Uehling, D.T., Wear, J.B., Gordon, E.S., Bargman, J.G., Deacon, J.S.R., Herrmann, J.P.R. and Opitz, J.M. (1975). Familial Kallmann syndrome with unilateral renal aplasia. *Clin. Genet.*, **7**, 368–81

27. Schopol, J., Mehltretter, G., von Zumbusch, R., Eversmann, T. and Von Werder, K. (1991). Comparison of gonadotrophin releasing hormone therapy in male patients with idiopathic hypothalamic hypogonadism. *Fertil. Steril.*, **56**, 1143–50

28. Liu, L., Banks, S., Barnes, K.M and Sherins, R.J. (1988). Two-year comparison of testicular responses to pulsatile gonadotrophin releasing hormone and exogenous gonadotrophins from the inception of therapy in men with isolated hypogonadotrophic hypogonadism. *J. Clin. Endocrinol. Metab.*, **67**, 1140–5

29. Kogan, S.J. (1987). Fertility in cryptorchidism. *Eur. J. Pediatr.*, **146**, S21–4

30. Gendrel, D., Roger, M. and Job, J.-C. (1980). Plasma gonadotropin and testosterone values in infants with cryptorchidism. *J. Paediatr.*, **97**, 217–20

31. Ley, S.B. and Leonard, J.M. (1985). Male hypogonadotrophic hypogonadism: factors influencing response to human chorionic gonadotrophin and human menopausal gonadotrophin, including prior exogenous androgens. *J. Clin. Endocrinol. Metab.*, **61**, 746–52

32. Mann, D.R., Gould, K.G., Collins, D.C. and Wallen, K. (1989). Blockade of neonatal activation of the pituitary testicular axis: effect of peripubertal luteinizing hormone and testosterone secretion and on testicular development in male monkeys. *J. Clin. Endocrinol. Metab.*, **68**, 600–7

33. Evain Brion, D., Gendrel, D., Bozzola, M., Chaussain, J. and Job, J.C. (1982). Diagnosis of Kallmann's syndrome in early infancy. *Acta Paediatr.*, **71**, 937–40

3

Pituitary destructive disorders

S. J. Holmes and S. M. Shalet

INTRODUCTION

Many patients with a mass lesion in the hypothalamic–pituitary area have reduced gonadotrophin secretion. The most common mass lesion in the pituitary fossa is a pituitary adenoma, and in the suprasellar region, a craniopharyngioma. There are several potential mechanisms for the reduced gonadotrophin secretion. A mass lesion within the pituitary fossa can interfere directly with pituitary gonadotrophin secretion and release. Alternatively, a mass lesion within the pituitary fossa or in the suprasellar area can interfere with hypothalamic secretion of gonadotrophin releasing hormone (GnRH) or its transport via the pituitary stalk, and hence cause gonadotrophin deficiency. Finally, hyperprolactinaemia suppresses the GnRH drive to the pituitary gonadotrophs causing gonadotrophin deficiency. Hyperprolactinaemia may be due to a prolactin-secreting adenoma, or to 'disconnection' from hypothalamic inhibitory control of prolactin secretion, due to a lesion affecting the hypothalamus or pituitary stalk. The recorded incidence of gonadotrophin deficiency in patients with untreated pituitary macroadenomas and suprasellar tumours is approximately 70–95%[1-4].

CUSHING'S DISEASE

Gonadotrophin deficiency has been demonstrated in patients with Cushing's disease[5-7]. Amenorrhoea or oligomenorrhoea has been reported to occur in approximately 75% of premenopausal women with Cushing's syndrome[8]. The pituitary adenoma in patients with Cushing's disease is usually very small (microadenoma), and does not cause sufficient destruction of pituitary tissue to interfere directly with gonadotrophin secretion, nor does it usually interfere directly with hypothalamic GnRH release and transport, or cause hyperprolactinaemia. The reduced gonadotrophin secretion in patients with Cushing's disease is instead thought to be partly due to suppression of gonadotrophin release by excess circulating glucocorticoids[6-8]. Gonadotrophin secretion tends to increase following successful treatment of Cushing's disease and restoration of normal concentrations of circulating glucocorticoids[6,7].

PITUITARY IRRADIATION

External irradiation of the hypothalamic–pituitary region for treatment of a pituitary adenoma or suprasellar tumour causes gonadotrophin deficiency[2,3,9]. Littley and colleagues[3] studied 165 patients who underwent external irradiation to the hypothalamic–pituitary region for treatment of a pituitary adenoma (84% of patients) or suprasellar tumour (16% of patients). A total of 140 patients had undergone pituitary surgery before radiotherapy. All patients received external irradiation with a dose of 3750–4250 cGy delivered in 15 or 16 fractions over 20–22 days. Before irradiation 79% of patients had gonadotrophin deficiency. Five years after irradiation 91% of the patients had abnormal gonadotrophin secretion; 8 years after irradiation 96% of the patients were gonadotrophin-deficient. This compares with 100% of patients having growth hormone (GH) deficiency 5 years after irradiation (82% deficient before irradiation), 84% of patients having adrenocorticotrophin (ACTH) deficiency 8 years after irradiation (41% deficient before irradiation) and 49% of patients having thyroid stimulating hormone (TSH) deficiency 8 years after irradiation (20% deficient before irradiation) (Figure 1).

In the patients who developed multiple pituitary hormone deficiencies following irradiation the most usual order of loss of anterior pituitary

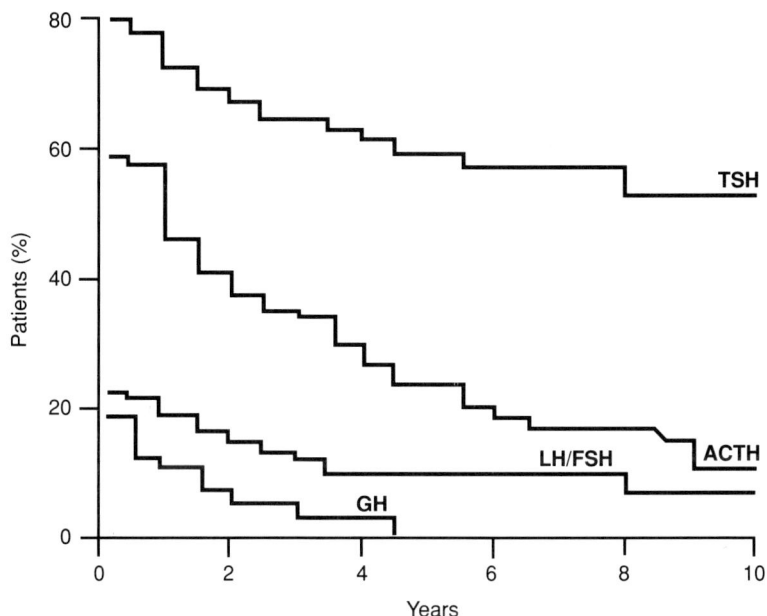

Figure 1 Cumulative percentages of patients with normal hypothalamic–pituitary–target gland axes plotted against time after radiotherapy

hormone function was GH followed by luteinizing hormone/follicle stimulating hormone (LH/FSH), ACTH and then TSH. This sequence was seen in 61% of the patients who developed multiple pituitary hormone deficiencies, although 25% of patients with non-functioning pituitary adenomas and 36% of patients with acromegaly who developed multiple deficiencies developed ACTH deficiency before LH/FSH deficiency. Snyder and associates[2] demonstrated that gonadotrophin deficiency developed in 50% of patients who had normal gonadotrophin secretion pretreatment, and who had not previously undergone pituitary surgery, 5 years following external pituitary irradiation at a dose of 4400–5000 cGy for treatment of a pituitary adenoma.

The development of gonadotrophin deficiency following external pituitary irradiation for treatment of pituitary disease is dose-dependent. Littley and co-workers[10] demonstrated that 5 years after irradiation the incidence of LH/FSH deficiency was 33% in patients with initially normal gonadotrophin secretion who received 2000 cGy delivered in eight fractions over 11 days. However, 66% of patients with previously normal gonadotrophin secretion developed LH/FSH deficiency 5 years after receiving 3500–4000 cGy delivered in 15 fractions over 21 days ($p < 0.05$). Total body irradiation for treatment of a haematological malignancy (1000 cGy in 5 fractions, or 1200 or 1320 cGy in 6 fractions, over 3 days) is associated with primary gonadal failure, but not with any damage to the hypothalamic–pituitary axis in the adult patient[11].

CRANIAL IRRADIATION

Cranial irradiation for treatment of a cranial tumour[12,13], tumours of the eye and middle ear[14] and nasopharyngeal carcinoma[15] can cause gonadotrophin deficiency, if the hypothalamic–pituitary axis lies within the radiation field. Lam and associates[15] demonstrated that gonadotrophin deficiency developed in 31% of adult patients 5 years after they received cranial irradiation at an estimated dose of 3980 cGy to the hypothalamus and 6170 cGy to the pituitary for treatment of nasopharyngeal carcinoma. However, 1 year after irradiation, men had a significant increase in basal levels of serum FSH, with no change in basal levels of serum LH and testosterone[16]. The integrated serum FSH response to LHRH was increased, while that of LH was decreased. From one year after irradiation there was a progressive decrease in stimulated serum LH, and in both basal and stimulated serum FSH. The authors propose that the fall in serum LH but rise in serum FSH in the first year following irradiation is due to a radiation-induced decrease in the pulse frequency of hypothalamic GnRH secretion. It has previously been proposed that the relative secretion rates of LH and FSH by the pituitary may be regulated by the frequency of pulsatile GnRH secretion from the hypothalamus[17,18], and a decreased LH pulse frequency (which suggests a decreased GnRH pulse frequency) has been demonstrated in men with selectively elevated serum FSH levels in the presence of normal serum LH levels[18]. The progressive decrease in secretion of both LH and FSH after the first year following irradiation[15] is in keeping with a progressive reduction in hypothalamic GnRH pulse amplitude[17].

HYPOTHALAMIC DAMAGE AND IRRADIATION

There are further observations that implicate the hypothalamus as the site of radiation-induced damage following irradiation of the hypothalamic–pituitary region. The peak serum LH and FSH responses to GnRH were delayed (gonadotrophin value at 60 min greater than that at 20 min) in subjects who developed gonadotrophin deficiency following hypothalamic–pituitary irradiation[3]. Serum LH showed a marked increase in response to GnRH but no increase in response to clomiphene, which is believed to increase hypothalamic secretion of GnRH, in women with irradiation-induced gonadotrophin deficiency[12]. In some subjects with radiation-induced GH deficiency, the peak serum GH response to a single bolus dose of GH releasing hormone was normal, but the peak serum GH response to the administration of arginine or to insulin-induced hypoglycaemia was reduced. Spontaneous secretion of GH may be reduced despite normal serum GH responses to pharmacological stimuli[19]. Finally, elevated serum prolactin levels following irradiation to the hypothalamic–pituitary axis[3] suggest damage to the hypothalamus.

PITUITARY GLAND SURGERY

Transsphenoidal surgery for removal of a pituitary adenoma may be complicated by removal of normally functioning pituitary tissue and hence gonadotrophin deficiency, or may cause recovery of previously suppressed gonadotrophin secretion, or may result in the gonadotrophin status of the patient remaining unchanged. Of patients who underwent transsphenoidal surgery for treatment of Cushing's disease or Nelson's syndrome, 48% acquired gonadotrophin deficiency postoperatively[20]. Of patients with gonadotrophin deficiency due to a non-functioning pituitary adenoma, 32% recovered gonadotrophin function following selective adenomectomy. The potential for recovery was related to the size of the adenoma before surgery and the severity of the pretreatment hypogonadism[1]. Gonadotrophin secretion was unchanged postoperatively in 89% of patients who underwent transsphenoidal surgery for treatment of a non-functioning pituitary adenoma[21]. The incidence of development of gonadotrophin deficiency depends on the amount of pituitary tissue removed at surgery. A radical procedure involving removal of all normal or doubtful tissue, with no visible normal gland left at the end of the operation, is associated with a greater occurrence of development of gonadotrophin deficiency than is a selective adenomectomy[20].

CYTOTOXIC DRUGS

Cytotoxic chemotherapy administered for treatment of haematological and other malignancies causes primary gonadal failure and hence hyper-gonadotrophic hypogonadism. There is no evidence to suggest that cytotoxic drugs have a direct action on the pituitary gonadotrophs.

THALASSAEMIA

It is well established that patients with β-thalassaemia major suffer from disorders of the hypothalamic–pituitary–gonadal axis, which are believed to result primarily from pituitary gonadotrophin insufficiency secondary to transfusional iron overload, in spite of treatment with the chelating agent desferrioxamine. The incidence of absence of any pubertal development in girls aged 12–18 years is 38%, with only 11% of girls under the age of 18 having experienced menarche[22]. The age at onset of menarche has been reported to be 2 years later than that of a control population[22,23]. The incidence of secondary amenorrhoea in transfusion-dependent thalassaemic subjects is reported to be between 35 and 100% in the 10 years following menarche[22,23]. Subjects with primary and secondary amenorrhoea have low basal levels of serum LH and FSH, and peak levels of serum LH and FSH after GnRH that are significantly lower than those in normal controls[23–25]. The pituitary gonadotrophin response to a bolus dose of GnRH does not increase following daily bolus doses of GnRH for 7 days prior to retesting[24], suggesting an abnormality in the pituitary gland or long-standing hypothalamic GnRH deficiency.

Further evidence for a pituitary abnormality was provided by Bergeron and Kovacs[26], who performed histological and immunocytological studies on pituitary glands of six patients with iron-overload states, including one patient with transfusional iron overload. They demonstrated a prefer-ential localization of iron in the gonadotrophs, compared with other anterior pituitary cells. In addition, Kletzky and colleagues[24] demonstrated haemosiderosis of the pituitary gland with no hypothalamic involvement at autopsy of an adult male with β-thalassaemia major. However, Chatterjee and associates[23] performed a prospective study of 15 girls with β-thalassaemia major, and found evidence to suggest a disturbance of hypothalamic GnRH secretion in addition to an abnormality of the pituitary gonadotrophs. All subjects had regular ovulatory menstrual cycles at the time of entry into the study, and all subsequently developed secondary amenorrhoea. The subjects underwent 12-hour gonadotrophin profiles, with blood samples taken every 15 min, and assessment of gonadotrophin responses to a bolus dose of GnRH before the onset of secondary amenorrhoea, and 12–14 months and 5–6 years after the onset of secondary amenorrhoea. While having regular menstrual cycles, the thalassaemic subjects had reduced pulsatile gonadotrophin secretion compared with control subjects, suggesting subtle damage to the hypothalamic GnRH pulse generator mechanism. The basal and GnRH-stimulated serum LH and FSH levels were lower in the patients than in the control subjects. Twelve to fourteen months after onset of amenorrhoea there were significant abnormalities in gonadotrophin pulse characteristics in all patients and a further reduction in GnRH-stimulated serum LH and FSH levels. By 5–6 years after the onset of amenorrhoea, 66% of patients had become apulsatile and had a further marked reduction in GnRH-stimulated gonadotrophin levels. These results suggest that there are abnormalities of the hypothalamic GnRH pulse-generating mechanism in addition to abnormalities of pituitary gonadotrophs in patients with β-thalassaemia major.

HAEMOCHROMATOSIS

Haemochromatosis can cause hypogonadism due to gonadotrophin deficiency, reported to occur in 17–75% of patients with haemo-chromatosis[27–31]. Gonadotrophin deficiency is believed to be due to iron deposition within the gonadotrophs of the pituitary gland, and possibly to a decrease in the number of pituitary gonadotrophs[26,32]. In the light of the work of Chatterjee and colleagues[23] in thalassaemic subjects, it is possible that haemochromatosis is associated with hypothalamic damage in addition to pituitary damage, thus leading to gonadotrophin deficiency. The propensity for haemochromatosis to damage the gonadotroph, but rarely other anterior pituitary cells, is not understood.

SHEEHAN'S SYNDROME

Sheehan's syndrome of postpartum pituitary necrosis is a cause of pituitary gonadotrophin deficiency. The serum LH response to a bolus dose of GnRH has been reported to be either reduced[33] or normal[34-36] in the majority of subjects with Sheehan's syndrome, and it has been proposed that the mechanism for the pituitary gonadotrophin deficiency involves the inability of hypothalamic GnRH to reach pituitary gonadotrophs[35]. Sheehan[37] observed that even when massive pituitary necrosis occurred, residual tissue remained at the pars tuberalis and in the two lateral poles of the pituitary gland. However, the lateral poles of the pituitary gland are not perfused by hypothalamic–hypophyseal portal blood and are therefore probably not exposed to hypothalamic GnRH. Nevertheless, endogenous pituitary gonadotrophin secretion may occasionally be normal in women with Sheehan's syndrome, as there are reports of successful pregnancies occurring in such women[38-41].

SARCOIDOSIS

Sarcoidosis can be associated with diffuse granulomatous infiltration of the hypothalamus, with little or no involvement of the pituitary gland. Granulomatous deposits in the region of the pituitary stalk can cause disconnection hyperprolactinaemia, with an increase in levels of serum prolactin reported to occur in up to one-third of patients with sarcoidosis. Gonadotrophin deficiency can occur as a consequence of the raised prolactin level[42] or may occur in the presence of normoprolactinaemia[43]. The responsiveness of serum LH and FSH to GnRH, but lack of response to clomiphene, indicates that diminished hypothalamic function is the major cause of the gonadotrophin deficiency[43].

HISTIOCYTOSIS X

Approximately one-third of patients with histiocytosis X have central diabetes insipidus as a consequence of histiocytic infiltration of the pituitary stalk and/or posterior pituitary gland. Very rarely, histiocytic infiltration of the hypothalamus or anterior pituitary gland can cause deficiencies of anterior pituitary hormones[44,45], including gonadotrophin deficiency, which is usually secondary to disconnection hyperprolactinaemia due to histiocytic infiltration of the hypothalamus and pituitary stalk[46].

LYMPHOCYTIC HYPOPHYSITIS

Lymphocytic hypophysitis is a rare disorder characterized by chronic inflammation within the pituitary gland and usually presents with features of hypopituitarism in young women in late pregnancy or in the postpartum period. Deficiency of pituitary gonadotrophins can occur secondarily to inflammatory infiltration of the anterior pituitary gland and subsequent destruction and fibrosis of pituitary tissue[47–49].

METASTASES TO THE PITUITARY GLAND

Metastases to the pituitary gland occur very rarely and are most commonly secondary to carcinoma of the breast in women and carcinoma of the bronchus in men[50,51]. Metastases occur more frequently to the posterior pituitary gland than the anterior pituitary gland[50,51], but can sometimes cause deficiencies of anterior pituitary hormones[52,53]. Pituitary metastases from renal cell carcinoma may present with features of hypo-pituitarism, including gonadotrophin deficiency, more frequently than do other metastatic tumours within the pituitary gland[54].

INFERTILITY TREATMENT

For those patients interested in fertility, it is of more than academic importance to determine if gonadotrophin deficiency associated with a destructive or infiltrative disorder is due to hypothalamic or to pituitary disease. Pulsatile GnRH therapy would only be suitable for patients with GnRH deficiency[55], but exogenous gonadotrophin therapy would be appropriate for any patient with gonadotrophin deficiency, irrespective of the site of damage.

REFERENCES

1. Arafah, B.M. (1986). Reversible hypopituitarism in patients with large non-functioning pituitary adenomas. *J. Clin. Endocrinol. Metab.*, **62**, 1173–9
2. Snyder, P.J., Fowble, B.F., Schatz, N.J., Savino, P.J. and Gennarelli, T.A. (1986). Hypopituitarism following radiation therapy of pituitary adenomas. *Am. J. Med.*, **81**, 457–62
3. Littley, M.D., Shalet, S.M., Beardwell, C.G., Ahmed, S.R., Applegate, G. and Sutton, M.L. (1989). Hypopituitarism following external radiotherapy for pituitary tumours in adults. *Q. J. Med.*, **70**, 145–60
4. Rivarola, M.A., Mendilaharzu, H., Warman, M., Belgorosky, A., Iorcansky, S., Castellano, M., Caresana, A., Chaler, E. and Maceiras, M. (1992). Endocrine disorders in 66 suprasellar and pineal tumors of patients with prepubertal and pubertal ages. *Horm. Res.*, **37**, 1–6
5. Boccuzzi, G., Angeli, A., Bisbocci, D., Fonzo, D., Gaidano, G.P. and Ceresa, F. (1975). Effect of synthetic luteinizing releasing hormone (LH-RH) on the release of gonadotrophins in Cushing's disease. *J. Clin. Endocrinol. Metab.*, **40**, 892–5
6. Luton, J.-P., Thieblot, P., Valcke, J.-C., Mahoudeau, J.A. and Bricaire, H. (1977). Reversible gonadotrophin deficiency in male Cushing's disease. *J. Clin. Endocrinol. Metab.*, **45**, 488–95
7. White, M.C., Sanderson, J., Mashiter, K. and Joplin, G.F. (1981). Gonadotrophin levels in women with Cushing's syndrome before and after treatment. *Clin. Endocrinol.*, **14**, 23–9
8. Aron, D.C., Schnall, A.M. and Sheeler, L.R. (1990). Cushing's syndrome and pregnancy. *Am. J. Obstet. Gynecol.*, **162**, 244–52
9. Feek, C.M., McLelland, J., Seth, J., Toft, A.D., Irvine, W.J., Padfield, P.L. and Edwards C.R.W. (1984). How effective is external pituitary irradiation for growth hormone-secreting pituitary tumours? *Clin. Endocrinol.*, **20**, 401–8
10. Littley, M.D., Shalet, S.M., Beardwell, C.G., Robinson, E.L. and Sutton, M.L. (1989). Radiation-induced hypopituitarism is dose-dependent. *Clin. Endocrinol.*, **31**, 363–73
11. Littley, M.D., Shalet, S.M., Morgenstern, G.R. and Deakin, D.P. (1991). Endocrine and reproductive dysfunction following fractionated total body irradiation in adults. *Q. J. Med.*, **78**, 265–74
12. Harrop, J.S., Davies, T.J., Capra, L.G. and Marks, V. (1976). Hypothalamic–pituitary function following successful treatment of intracranial tumours. *Clin. Endocrinol.*, **5**, 313–21
13. Constine, L.S., Woolf, P.D., Cann, D., Mick, G., McCormick, K., Raubertas, R.F. and Rubin, P. (1993). Hypothalamic–pituitary dysfunction after radiation for brain tumors. *N. Engl. J. Med.*, **328**, 87–94

14. Richards, G.E., Wara, W.M., Grumbach, M.M., Kaplan, S.L., Sheline, G.E. and Conte, F.A. (1976). Delayed onset of hypopituitarism: sequelae of therapeutic irradiation of central nervous system, eye, and middle ear tumors. *J. Paediatr.*, **89**, 553–9

15. Lam, K.S.L., Tse, V.K.C., Wang, C., Yeung, R.T.T. and Ho, J.H.C. (1991). Effects of cranial irradiation on hypothalamic-pituitary function – a 5-year longitudinal study in patients with nasopharyngeal carcinoma. *Q. J. Med.*, **78**, 165–76

16. Lam, K.S.L., Tse, V.K.C., Wang, C., Yeung, R.T.T., Ma, J.T.C. and Ho, J.H.C. (1987). Early effects of cranial irradiation on hypothalamic-pituitary function. *J. Clin. Endocrinol. Metab.*, **64**, 418–24

17. Wildt, L., Hausler, A., Marshall, G., Hutchison, J.S., Plant, T.M., Belchetz, P.E. and Knobil, E. (1981). Frequency and amplitude of gonadotrophin-releasing hormone stimulation and gonadotrophin secretion in the Rhesus monkey. *Endocrinology*, **109**, 376–85

18. Gross, K.M., Matsumoto, A.M., Southworth, M.B. and Bremner, W.J. (1985). Evidence for decreased luteinizing hormone-releasing hormone pulse frequency in men with selective elevations of follicle-stimulating hormone. *J. Clin. Endocrinol. Metab.*, **60**,197–202

19. Shalet, S.M. (1993). Radiation and pituitary dysfunction. *N. Engl. J. Med.*, **328**, 131–3

20. Burke, C.W., Adams, C.B.T., Esiri, M.M., Morris, C. and Bevan, J.S. (1990). Transsphenoidal surgery for Cushing's disease: does what is removed determine the endocrine outcome? *Clin. Endocrinol.*, **33**, 525–37

21. Comtois, R., Beauregard, H., Somma, M., Serri, O., Aris-Jilwan, N. and Hardy, J. (1991). The clinical and endocrine outcome to trans-sphenoidal microsurgery of nonsecreting pituitary adenomas. *Cancer*, **68**, 860–6

22. Borgna-Pignatti, C., De Stefano, P., Zonta, L., Vullo, C., De Sanctis, V., Melevendi, C., Naselli, A., Masera, G., Terzoli, S., Gabutti, V. and Piga, A. (1985). Growth and sexual maturation in thalassaemia major. *J. Paediatr.*, **106**, 150–5

23. Chatterjee, R., Katz, M., Cox, T.F. and Porter, J.B. (1993). Prospective study of the hypothalamic-pituitary axis in thalassaemic patients who developed secondary amenorrhoea. *Clin. Endocrinol.*, **39**, 287–96

24. Kletzky, O.A., Costin, G., Marrs, R., Bernstein, G., March, C.M. and Mishell, D.R. (1979). Gonadotrophin insufficiency in patients with thalassaemia major. *J. Clin. Endocrinol. Metab.*, **48**, 901–5

25. De Sanctis, V., Vullo, C., Katz, M., Wonke, B., Hoffbrand, A.V. and Bagni, B. (1988). Hypothalamic–pituitary–gonadal axis in thalassaemic patients with secondary amenorrhoea. *Obstet. Gynecol.*, **72**, 643–7

26. Bergeron, C. and Kovacs, K. (1978). Pituitary siderosis: a histologic,

immunocytologic, and ultrastructural study. *Am. J. Pathol.*, **93**, 295–310

27. Stocks, A.E. and Powell, L.W. (1972). Pituitary function in idiopathic haemochromatosis and cirrhosis of the liver. *Lancet*, **2**, 298–300

28. Walsh, C.H., Wright, A.D., Williams, J.W. and Holder, G. (1976). A study of pituitary function in patients with idiopathic haemochromatosis. *J. Clin. Endocrinol. Metab.*, **43**, 866–72

29. Bezwoda, W.R., Bothwell, T.H., Van Der Walt, L.A., Kronheim, S. and Pimstone, B.L. (1977). An investigation into gonadal dysfunction in patients with idiopathic haemochromatosis. *Clin. Endocrinol.*, **6**, 377–85

30. Charbonnel, B., Chupin, M., LeGrand, A. and Guillon, J. (1981). Pituitary function in idiopathic haemochromatosis: hormonal study in 36 male patients. *Acta Endocrinol.*, **98**, 178–83

31. Walton, C., Kelly, W.F., Laing, I. and Bullock, D.E. (1983). Endocrine abnormalities in idiopathic haemochromatosis. *Q. J. Med.*, **205**, 99–110

32. MacDonald, R.A. and Mallory, G.K. (1960). Haemochromatosis and haemosiderosis. *Arch. Int. Med.*, **105**, 686–700

33. Aono, T., Minagawa, J., Kinugasa, T., Tanizawa, O. and Kurachi, K. (1973). Response of pituitary LH and FSH to synthetic LH-releasing hormone in normal subjects and patients with Sheehan's syndrome. *Am. J. Obstet. Gynecol.*, **117**, 1046–52

34. Mortimer, R.H., Fleischer, N., Lev-Gur, M. and Freeman, R.G. (1976). Correlation between integrated LH and FSH levels and the response to luteinizing hormone releasing factor (LRF). *J. Clin. Endocrinol. Metab.*, **43**, 1240–9

35. Shahmanesh, M., Ali, Z., Pourmand, M. and Nourmand, I. (1980). Pituitary function in Sheehan's syndrome. *Clin. Endocrinol.*, **12**, 303–11

36. Jialal, I., Naidoom C., Norman, R.J., Rajput, M.C., Omar, M.A.K. and Joubert, S.M. (1984). Pituitary function in Sheehan's syndrome. *Obstet. Gynecol.*, **63**, 15–19

37. Sheehan, H.L. (1961). Atypical hypopituitarism. *Proc. R. Soc. Med.*, **54**, 43–8

38. Jackson, I.M., Whyte, W.G. and Garrey, M.M. (1969). Pituitary function following uncomplicated pregnancy in Sheehan's syndrome. *J. Clin. Endocrinol. Metab.*, **29**, 315–18

39. Martin, J.E., MacDonald, P.C. and Kaplan, N.M. (1970). Successful pregnancy in a patient with Sheehan's syndrome. *N. Engl. J. Med.*, **282**, 425–7

40. Moreira, A.C., Maciel, L.M., Foss, M.C., Verissimo, J.M.T. and Iazigi, N. (1984). Gonadotrophin secretory capacity in a patient with Sheehan's syndrome with successful pregnancies. *Fertil. Steril.*, **42**, 303–5

41. Grimes, H.G. and Brooks, M.H. (1980). Pregnancy in Sheehan's syndrome. Report of a case and review. *Obstet. Gynecol. Surv.*, **35**, 481–8

42. Lawton, F.G., Shalet, S.M., Beardwell, C.G. and Daws, R.A. (1982). Hypothalamic–pituitary disease as the sole manifestation of sarcoidosis. *Postgrad. Med. J.*, **58**, 771–2

43. Stuart, C.A., Neelon, F.A. and Lebovitz, H.E. (1978). Hypothalamic insufficiency: the cause of hypopituitarism in sarcoidosis. *Ann. Intern. Med.*, **88**, 589–94

44. Braunstein, G.D. and Kohler, P.O. (1972). Pituitary function in Hand–Schüller–Christian disease. *N. Engl. J. Med.*, **286**, 1225–9

45. Pressman, B.D., Waldron, R.L. II and Wood, E.H. (1975). Histiocytosis-X of the hypothalamus. *Br. J. Radiol.*, **48**, 176–8

46. Gates, R.B., Friesen, H. and Samaan, N.A. (1973). Inappropriate lactation and amenorrhoea: pathological and diagnostic considerations. *Acta Endocrinol.*, **72**, 101–14

47. Guay, A.T., Agnello, V., Tronic, B.C., Gresham, D.G. and Freidberg, S.R. (1987). Lymphocytic hypophysitis in a man. *J. Clin. Endocrinol. Metab.*, **64**, 631–4

48. Cosman, F., Post, K.D., Holub, D.A. and Wardlaw, S.L. (1989). Lymphocytic hypophysitis. Report of 3 new cases and review of the literature. *Med. Baltimore*, **68**, 240–56

49. Pestell, R.G., Best, J.D. and Alford, F.P. (1990). Lymphocytic hypophysitis. The clinical spectrum of the disorder and evidence for an autoimmune pathogenesis. *Clin. Endocrinol.*, **33**, 457–66

50. Kovacs K. (1973). Metastatic cancer of the pituitary gland. *Oncology*, **27**, 533–42

51. Teears, R.J. and Silverman, E.M. (1975). Clinicopathologic review of 88 cases of carcinoma metastatic to the pituitary gland. *Cancer*, **36**, 216–20

52. Epstein, S., Ranchod, M. and Goldswain, P.R.T. (1973). Pituitary insufficiency, inappropriate antidiuretic hormone (ADH) secretion, and carcinoma of the bronchus. *Cancer*, **32**, 476–81

53. Branch, C.L. and Laws, E.R. (1987). Metastatic tumors of the sella turcica masquerading as primary pituitary tumors. *J. Clin. Endocrinol. Metab.*, **65**, 469–74

54. Koshiyama, H., Ohgaki, K., Hida, S., Takasu, K., Yumitori, K., Shimatsu, A. and Koh, T. (1992). Metastatic renal cell carcinoma to the pituitary gland presenting with hypopituitarism. *J. Endocrinol. Invest.*, **15**, 677–81

55. Morris, D.V., Abdulwahid, N.A., Armar, A. and Jacobs, H.S. (1987). The response of patients with organic hypothalamic–pituitary disease to pulsatile gonadotrophin-releasing hormone therapy. *Fertil. Steril.*, **47**, 54–9

4

Disorders of puberty

S. L. B. Duncan

INTRODUCTION

In the transition of a girl to full sexual maturity, growth and development are very variable with much overlap between normal and abnormal. Special sensitivities arise when there are problems. She may have difficulty expressing her anxieties, and embarrassment or uncertainty about her physical changes, yet this may also be the time when she is beginning to seek advice on her own. Consistency of medical advice is very important, yet it is also often the time of change from paediatrician to adult physician. Any shortcomings of trust at this time may cast a long shadow into the future.

Endocrinological and gynaecological aspects of puberty have to be set into the context of paediatric gynaecology. Some conditions recognized at birth or in early life, for example Turner's or adrenogenital syndrome, have special needs around the time of puberty. The recognition of precocious or delayed puberty rests essentially on timing. Yet others, for example hirsutism or anomalous development, are liable to develop at puberty and may cause consternation.

Although the main focus of this section is on endocrine aspects of puberty, the identification of anatomical problems is recognized to be important in differentiation.

CONTROL OF NORMAL PUBERTY

The endocrine mechanisms are in place from foetal life. In particular, the hypothalamus and pituitary are active in foetal and early neonatal life and then become suppressed. Some ovarian activity continues during childhood.

The events of maturation are complex and involve thyroid and adrenal glands as well as nutritional and psychological states. The essential hormonal event of adolescence is augmentation of pulsatile gonadotrophin secretion. This, in turn, is associated with increased pituitary sensitivity to gonadotrophin releasing hormone (GnRH) and also with increased ovarian sensitivity to the gonadotrophin pulses. Rosenfield provides a useful review of this topic[1].

There are good cross-sectional and longitudinal data about somatic growth and puberty development in many populations, with wide agreement about the average sequence and intervals. Standards for girls in the UK are generally based on the work of Marshall and Tanner[2]. The growth spurt is intrinsically linked to increasing oestrogen levels and is detectable just before the earliest breast bud changes.

Ovarian and uterine changes

Ultrasound has greatly extended our appreciation of ovarian and uterine growth in normal girls. The ovaries are not quiescent in childhood but often contain functional microcysts even from an early age[3]. As the ovaries mature there is a very slight increase of size with increasing age[4] and this increase seems to be due more to an increase in the proportion of multicystic ovaries than to any relation to hormone levels. Within the pubertal period significant enlargement of the ovaries occurs only after breast stage 3[3].

Uterine size does not appear to increase materially from age 2 until about age 7 and from then on, there is age-related growth, with a relative increase in the corpus[3]. Once pubertal development has started, an increase in uterine size is related to oestradiol stimulation. The main differential increase in relation to body size seems to occur between breast stages 3 and 4[3]. Inhibin levels rise steeply between breast stages 2 and 4[5].

It is generally just after breast stage 4, when enough endometrium has grown in response to the oestrogen stimulation, that withdrawal bleeding occurs as a result of a cyclical fall in oestrogens. Thus, of itself, menarche is not a hormonally significant event, but its occurrence denotes some development in cyclical pituitary–ovarian activity, although the initial cycles are rarely ovulatory. Because it can be dated and later recalled, it becomes an event of some significance. Its timing usually denotes the late stages of the growth period.

Controlling influences

Factors which influence the onset and rate of these changes include nutrition, physical activity, urbanization and genetic influences. Uncertainties, however, remain. There is some evidence in a recent anthropomorphic study from Holland[6] that later onset of puberty is associated with faster progress – a concept of 'catch-up' pubertal maturation.

DISORDERED PUBERTY

It is the variability about the mean which provides the standards for the definition of precocious and delayed puberty. Within even the normal time-scale, puberty sequence may be disordered, arrested or anomalous. Only examples of precocious and delayed puberty are referred to in this contribution.

Investigation of disordered puberty consists essentially of assessing the present puberty status and consideration of appropriate possible causes. Management often hinges on the objectives to be achieved rather than on the underlying diagnosis.

Precocious puberty

Precocious puberty is usually defined as breast development before 8 years, pubic hair before 8.5 years or menses before 9.5 years, each of which is more than 2 standard deviations before the mean age. The diagnostic challenge is to establish whether specific features are isolated or part of a co-ordinated disturbance. Basic causes can be central or peripheral (Table 1).

Table 1 Main causes of precocious puberty

Type	Cause
Central (true)	CNS tumour, especially hypothalamic, hamartoma CNS disorder, e.g. post-encephalitis, hydrocephaly hypothyroidism idiopathic
Peripheral	ovarian adrenal – adrenogenital syndrome McCune–Albright syndrome
Exogenous	oestrogens androgens
Variants	premature thelarche or adrenarche

Table 2 Features of precocious puberty

Acceleration in height	Sensitivity to GnRH
Advanced skeletal age	Increased ovarian size
Pubertal luteinizing hormone and follicle stimulating hormone	Increased uterine size
Pubertal oestradiol	

The younger the girl, the greater is the problem and the more important must be the search for disorders of the central nervous system. The investigation essentially hinges on the search for normal pubertal events at an inappropriate age (Table 2).

In idiopathic precocious puberty, which is the commonest diagnosis in this condition, the ovaries and uterus are enlarged to a size consonant with that of puberty[4]. This is predominantly due to an exaggeration of the multicystic appearance common in childhood. Interestingly, individual follicle size is not usually increased[4].

Removal or treatment of a peripheral, exogenous or central nervous system cause is indicated, where this is appropriate. In central, idiopathic precocious puberty, GnRH analogues are highly effective with regression of ovarian and uterine size and of secondary sexual characteristics.

Table 3 Main causes of delayed puberty

Manifestation	Cause
Little or no evidence of gonadal function (age 13 onwards)	
Hypergonadotrophin	ovarian failure ± abnormal chromosomes
Hypogonadotrophin reversible	thyroid weight-related constitutional
irreversible	pituitary deficiency congenital CNS defects
Evidence of gonadal function (age 15 onwards or 3 years since start of breast development)	
Anatomic defect	agenesis obstruction
Anovulation	inappropriate feedback androgen insensitivity or variant

Long-term follow-up of idiopathic precocious puberty has previously been reasssuring[7] in terms of menstrual function and fertility, although restriction of height has been common. Follow-up after GnRH agonists is still limited, but is encouraging with respect to deceleration of bone age and a subsequent increase in predicted adult height[8]. In a study of up to 7 years' follow-up after the onset of treatment, there has been a high rate of ovulation (about 90%) in girls studied at least 2 years after menarche[9].

Delayed puberty

It is obvious, from consideration of the puberty maturation processes and from the wide variety of possible causes (Table 3), that a single chronological age is not an adequate alert signal for diagnosis. Short stature should prompt investigation sooner than delay in the onset of pubertal changes, which, in turn, should arouse anxiety at an earlier age than failure of menarche. Anomalous development requires a sympathetic response when any anxiety is aroused. Systematic consideration of the puberty status, search for evidence of other endocrine disorders and observation for changes over a period will narrow down the diagnostic possibilities. The presence or absence of evidence of ovarian function is a fundamental differentiating feature. In practice, one of the residual difficulties is the differentiation between hypogonadotrophic hypo-thalamic causes and constitutional delay. Either may be partial and present as arrest of development. Management depends on whether short stature is a feature and on the stage of epiphyseal closure. Growth hormone (GH) and/or low doses of oestrogen will allow an increase in stature to precede a controlled rate of development of secondary characteristics. Final differentiation may have to await study of the response to withdrawal of oestrogen replacement. GnRH can be used in a pulsatile fashion[10] but this is inconvenient and expensive, necessarily prolonged and is very intrusive in a teenage life-style.

Turner's syndrome

Earlier diagnosis, often in response to short stature, makes Turner's syndrome more of a paediatric problem at present, with treatment for growth preceding that for puberty development There are intrinsic somatic and skeletal as well as hormonal aspects but lack of ovarian production of oestrogens in childhood reduces pituitary feedback. Follicle stimulating hormone (FSH) is raised at an earlier age. There is failure of the normal boost that oestradiol production provides to the secretion of GH and insulin–like growth factor (IGF–I) and which is most evident during the phase of rapid growth[11]. In the natural history of the condition there is no growth spurt but there is longer than usual continued growth. Growth hormone, oestrogens and oxandrolone each cause a growth spurt provided they are given before epiphyseal closure (Figure 1). The current aims of management are clear (Table 4) although optimum timing and dose regimes are still a matter for study. Until recently, oestrogens have been introduced early (e.g. from age 10) in very low doses to achieve a growth spurt without undue skeletal maturation. The dosage used has been:

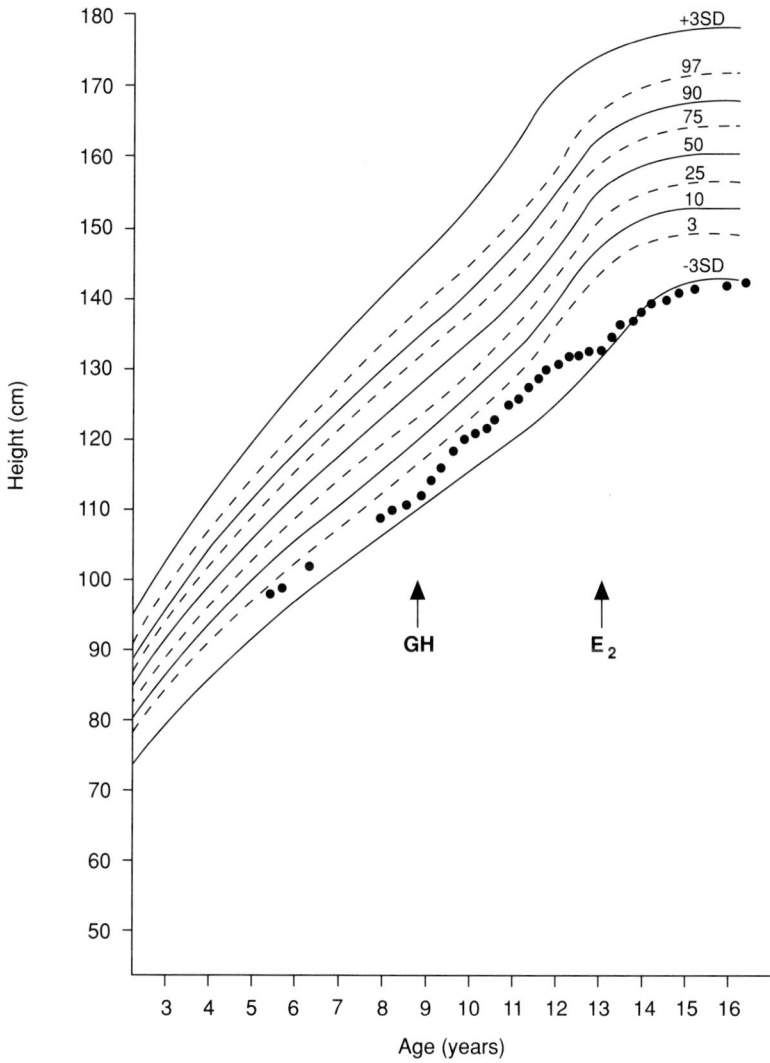

Figure 1 Growth chart of a girl with Turner's syndrome, showing a growth spurt in response to growth hormone (GH) and a later one in response to oestradiol (E_2), with continued slight growth but restricted final height

1st year:	2–5 µg/day(i.e. 50–100 ng/kg/day)
2nd year:	5–10 µg/day (i.e. 100–200 ng/kg/day)
3rd year:	10–20 µg/day

These increments are achieved according to response and the aim is to reach withdrawal bleeds (usually requiring 20 µg/day given with a week's break) by about 13 years. A combined oestrogen–progestogen preparation is then introduced for long-term use. However, where diagnosis is early enough, the use of GH is encouraging. Several short-term studies[12] have shown that GH accelerates growth with net gain in height, compared with previous standards, despite some acceleration of skeletal maturation. A long-term multicentre study with a mean age of start of GH treatment of 9.3 years (range 4.7–12.4)[13] provides encouraging results. Maximum growth rate occurs in the first 2 years of treatment but sustained growth for 6 years has occurred with appreciable increase of actual compared with predicted height. The additional benefit of oxandrolone seems to be marginal. Where GH can be given timely to achieve increase in height without risk of premature puberty development, the slow prolonged administration of oestrogens may become less crucial and a start age of about 11 or 12 years with slightly faster progression may become more appropriate. At the moment, the plan should either be part of a planned trial or be highly individualized.

It is not yet certain that final height in women with Turner's syndrome will be influenced, but the attainment of milestones at closer to the normal range is of obvious benefit. Early diagnosis and intervention is essential to achieve this. The possibility of donor egg pregnancy has revolutionized counselling and outlook.

Table 4 Aims of management in Turner's syndrome

Avoid acceleration of bone age

Minimize height deficit compared with peer group

Promote secondary sex characteristics at the average age

Attend to psychosocial aspects

Table 5 Gynaecological and puberty problems in adrenogenital syndrome

---

Gynaecological aspects

Amenorrhoea (primary or secondary)
Apareunia
Infertility
Pregnancy

Puberty

Development frequently disordered
Adrenarche early
Height restricted
Breast development variable in timing
Menarche apt to be late (or never)
Highly variable problem of pelvic anatomy

Adrenogenital syndrome

In adrenogenital syndrome, there are significant problems at puberty. In general, where the condition is of the salt-losing type, there is a more severe enzyme defect and more severe *in utero* fusion of the lower genital tract.

In the last generation or so, more such girls have survived into adulthood. Gynaecological and puberty problems are common (Table 5). In practice, adult height tends to be below average. In one large study of women[14], the mean final adult height of 40 women with simple virilizing congenital adrenal hyperplasia was 153.3 cm, and in 40 women with the salt-losing form, it was 156.8 cm, approximating to the 10th and 25th centiles, respectively, for normal women. It seems likely that the slight but significant difference between these groups is due to greater treatment compliance in early years in the salt-losing group necessitated by their condition rather than to an intrinsic differential biological effect.

The sequence of puberty development may be disordered because adrenarche, which exerts a somewhat independent influence, is more likely to be advanced or unusually inhibited (due to treatment) and likewise, growth is less closely related to ovarian oestrogens than usual (Figure 2). Certainly, bone age seems to be much less closely related to

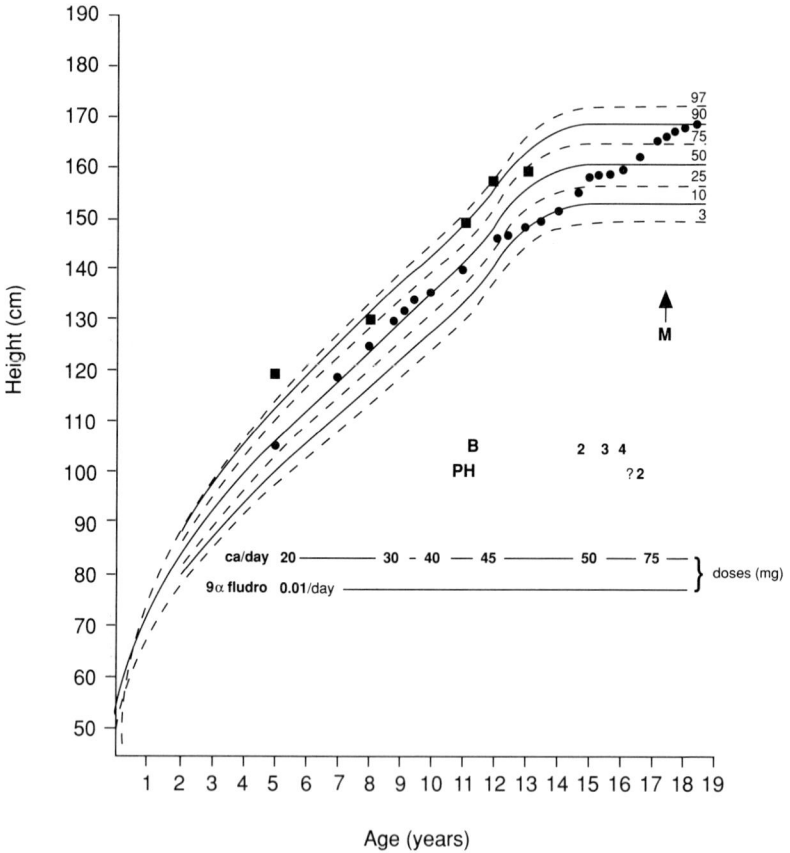

Figure 2 Growth and development chart of a girl with adrenogenital syndrome, showing interruption of prolonged growth spurt, and discrepancy between bone and chronological age and late menarche. B, breast stage; PH, pubic hair; M, menarche; ca, cortisone acetate; 9α fludro, 9α fludrocortisone

menarche, which is often delayed, even with apparently good control. Beyond puberty, oligomenorrhoea and anovulation are common and fertility is apt to be impaired. Ovulatory disorders prove to be particularly difficult to remedy. There is a very variable problem of genital anatomy.

The need for and complexity of vaginal surgery is affected both by the severity of the enzyme defect and by any surgery in early life.

It is not certain whether good replacement therapy over the early years will affect the onset of menarche or fertility, but perhaps the simplest index of this will be final height and the spontaneous onset of menses.

PRACTICAL SCHEME FOR CONSIDERATION OF DELAY IN PUBERTY MATURATION

In practice, most healthy girls go through puberty development normally, albeit at different times and rates. The incidence of major problems is low. The first contact because of anxiety is generally made with a primary practitioner, who will see many more variants of the normal compared with serious problems. It follows that the girl with the occasional important abnormality is often first seen by a practitioner unfamiliar with the problem and reassurance may lead to inappropriate delay. On the other hand, premature investigation is likely to lead to unnecessary anxiety and wasteful use of resources. Short stature is often ignored until there is recognition of delay of secondary sex characteristics. Complicating medical problems, e.g. diabetes, asthma and thyroid problems, may be under-diagnosed, or recognized and adduced as the cause of the delayed onset of puberty.

Menarche is apt to be awaited long after the appropriate growth and breast development, and the problem of obstructed menses may be diagnosed unnecessarily late. Conversely, it is not appropriate to expect menarche unless there has been a growth spurt and breast development to stage 4.

A simple, practical 'first-line' scheme has therefore been devised (Figure 3) to provide a rational starting point. This is based on mean ages of the key events and their relative time-scale so that the pattern can be followed, regardless of actual chronological age.

Delay matters:

(1) If there is short stature;

(2) If there is systemic disease, e.g. hypothyroidism or diabetes, needing management;

(3) If there are virilizing features; and

(4) If there is menstrual obstruction.

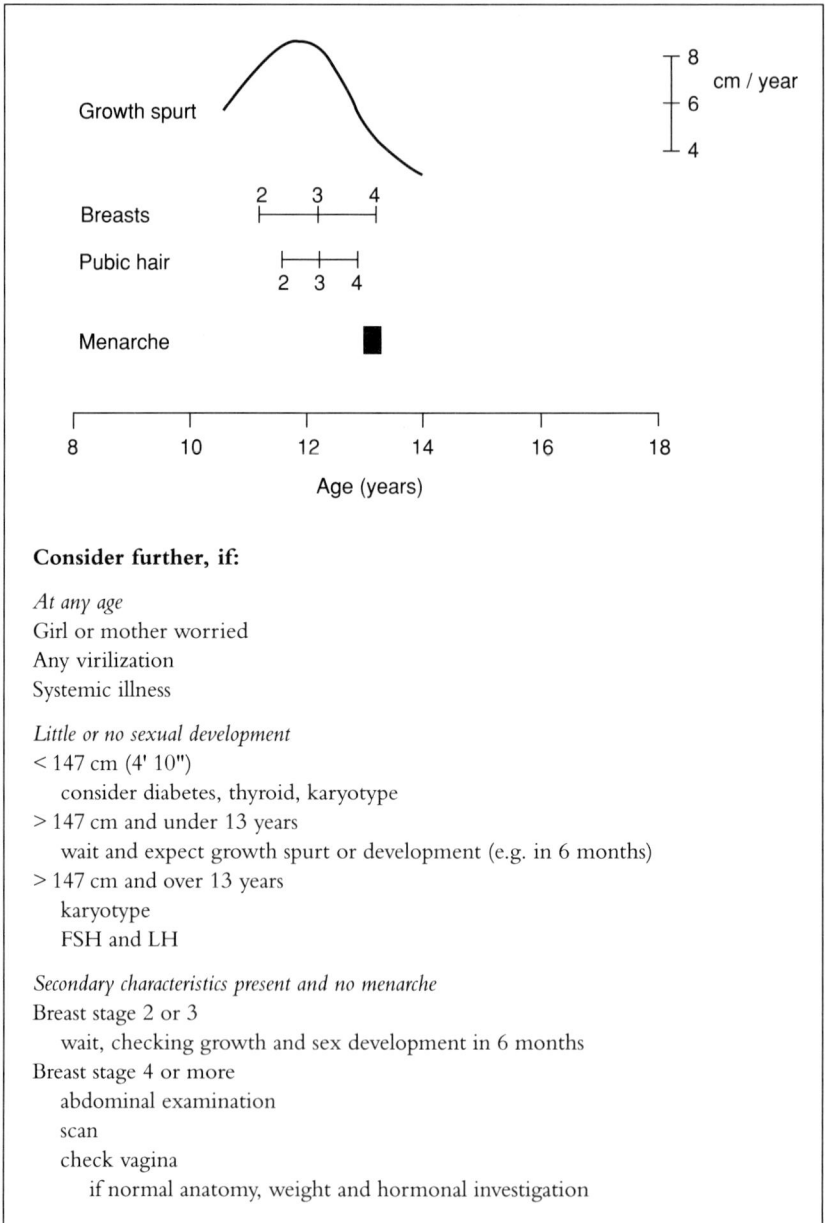

Consider further, if:

At any age
Girl or mother worried
Any virilization
Systemic illness

Little or no sexual development
< 147 cm (4' 10")
    consider diabetes, thyroid, karyotype
> 147 cm and under 13 years
    wait and expect growth spurt or development (e.g. in 6 months)
> 147 cm and over 13 years
    karyotype
    FSH and LH

Secondary characteristics present and no menarche
Breast stage 2 or 3
    wait, checking growth and sex development in 6 months
Breast stage 4 or more
    abdominal examination
    scan
    check vagina
        if normal anatomy, weight and hormonal investigation

Figure 3 Suggested basic scheme for primary care, if there is anxiety about puberty development

Otherwise, observation of progress over a short (e.g. 6-month) period will be more appropriate, to spot the occasional anomaly.

Essentially, therefore:

(1) If there is anxiety about lack of onset of sexual development, the priority is to consider systemic disorders and causes of short stature.

(2) By 13 years, at any height, absence of breast development is outside normality and should be investigated.

(3) If there is some puberty development, serial observation is appropriate until there is arrest or achievement of breast stage 4 for 6 months, in which case referral should be made.

REFERENCES

1. Rosenfield, R.L. (1991). Puberty and its disorders in girls. *Endocrinol. Metab. Clin. N. Am.*, **20**, 15–41
2. Marshall, W.A. and Tanner, J.M. (1969). Variations in patterns of pubertal changes in girls. *Arch. Dis. Child.*, **44**, 291–303
3. Salardi, S., Orsini, L.F., Cacciari, E., Bovicelli, L., Tassoni, P. and Reggiani, A. (1985). Pelvic ultrasonography in pre-menarchial girls: relation to puberty and sex hormone concentrations. *Arch. Dis. Child.*, **60**, 120–5
4. Stanhope, R., Adams, J., Jacobs, H.S. and Brook, C.G.D. (1985). Ovarian ultrasound assessment in normal children, idiopathic precocious puberty, and during low dose pulsatile gonadotrophin releasing hormone treatment of hypogonadotrophin hypogonadism. *Arch. Dis. Child.*, **60**, 116–19
5. Burger, H.G., McLachlan, R.I., Bangah, M., Quigg, H., Findlay, J.K., Robertson, D.M., De Kretser, D.M., Warne, G.L., Werther, G.A., Hudson, I.L., Cook, J.J., Fiedler, R., Greco, S., Yong, A.B.W. and Smith, P. (1988). Serum inhibin concentrations rise throughout normal male and female puberty. *J. Clin. Endocrinol. Metab.*, **76**, 689–94
6. de Ridder, C.M., Thijssen, J.H.H., Bruning, P.F., Van den Brande, J.L., Zonderland, M.L. and Erich, W.B.M. (1992). Body fat mass, body fat distribution, and pubertal development: a longitudinal study of physical and hormonal sexual maturation of girls. *J. Clin. Endocrinol. Metab.* **75**, 442–6
7. Murran, D., Dewhurst, J. and Grant, D.B. (1984). Precocious puberty: a follow-up study. *Arch. Dis. Child.*, **59**, 77–8
8. Swaenpoel, C., Chaussain, J.L. and Roger, M. (1991). Long-term results of long-acting luteinizing-hormone-releasing hormone agonist in central precocious puberty. *Horm. Res.*, **36**, 126–30

9. Jay, N., Mansfield, M.J., Blizzard, R.M., Crowley, W.F. Jr, Schoenfeld, D., Rhubin, L. and Boepple, P.A. (1992). Ovulation and menstrual function of adolescent girls with central precocious puberty after therapy with gonadotrophin-releasing hormone agonists. *J. Clin. Endocrinol. Metab.*, **75**, 890–4

10. Stanhope, R., Brook, C.G.D., Pringle, P.J., Adams, J. and Jacobs, H.S. (1987). Induction of puberty by pulsatile gonadotrophin releasing hormone. *Lancet,* **2**, 552–5

11. Rogol, A.D. (1992). Growth and growth hormone secretion at puberty: the role of gonadal steroid hormones. *Acta Paediatr.* (Suppl.) **383**, 15–20

12. Takano, K., Hizuka, N. and Shizume, K. (1986). Growth hormone treatment in Turner's syndrome. *Acta Paediatr.* (Suppl.) **325**, 58–63

13. Rosenfield, R.G. and the Genentech National Co-operative Study Group (1992). Growth hormone therapy in Turner's syndrome: an update on final height. *Acta. Paediatr.* (Suppl.), **383**, 3–6

14. Mulaikal, R.M., Migeon, C.J. and Rock, J.A. (1987). Fertility rates in female patients with congenital adrenal hyperplasia due to 21-hydroxylase deficiency. *N. Engl. J. Med.*, **316**, 178–82

5

Psychoneuroendocrinology

M. C. White

INTRODUCTION

Psychoneuroendocrinology is the study of the effects of higher brain function on the endocrine system. The natural circadian rhythms of hormone secretion are examples of cortical influence on otherwise closed endocrine feedback loops, as illustrated by the early morning rise of adrenocorticotrophin (ACTH) and cortisol, the regular evening rise of thyroid stimulating hormone, and the episodic release of growth hormone which occurs during sleep. Alterations in photoperiodicity, largely reflected in the change from winter to summer, also affect hormonal function[1], and presumably do so through cortical brain pathways.

CENTRAL CONTROL MECHANISMS AFFECTING GONADOTROPHIN RELEASING HORMONE RELEASE

Normal gonadal function in the female is dependent on a regular but changeable, cyclical, pulsatile secretion of gonadotrophin releasing hormone (GnRH) which controls the release of pituitary gonadotrophins, predominantly luteinizing hormone (LH). Interruption of the normal regulation of GnRH secretion will result in oligo- or amenorrhoea and/or anovulation. The spontaneous pulsatile secretion of GnRH is influenced by many different neurotransmitters and is modulated by ovarian sex steroids and possibly other ovarian peptides. Catecholamines, adrenaline and noradrenaline and vasoactive intestinal peptide are stimulatory, whereas opioid peptides, γ-aminobutyric acid and corticotrophin releasing factor (CRF) are inhibitory. Neuropeptide Y (NPY), dopamine and serotonin can have both stimulatory and inhibitory effects.

The LH pulse frequency in the luteal phase of normal cycling females is influenced by an inhibitory action of progesterone on the hypothalamic release of GnRH. This effect can be reversed by the administration of opiate antagonists such as naloxone[2]. Such drugs will also enhance LH pulsatility and amplitude in the late follicular phase of the cycle but not in the early follicular phase, when oestradiol levels are much lower[2,3]. Thus there is good physiological evidence that opiates modulate the pattern of GnRH pulsatility during the latter half of the menstrual cycle, and clearly a change in central opioidergic activity could be of relevance to pathological states causing oligo- or amenorrhoea. Dopamine appears to have a small physiological effect on LH release in the normal cycle, and this is mainly inhibitory, occurring in the late follicular phase[4].

GONADOTROPHIN REGULATION IN CENTRAL DISORDERS OF MENSTRUATION

Recognized clinical conditions which are associated with ovarian dysfunction due to the disruption of GnRH pulsatility and secretion include 'stress–related' amenorrhoea, hypothalamic amenorrhoea and anorexia nervosa. Many would consider that 'stress–related' and hypothalamic amenorrhoea are the same condition. Hypothalamic dysregulation has also been proposed as a cause of the polycystic ovary syndrome, but the evidence for this remains very tenuous[5].

In women with hypothalamic amenorrhoea, LH pulse frequency is most commonly akin to that seen in the late luteal phase of the normal menstrual cycle, but oestradiol levels are lower and follicle stimulating hormone levels higher. The key feature is an unchanging cyclical gonadotrophin secretion which appears to result from a decreased frequency and amplitude of GnRH pulsatile secretion, and thus a decreased stimulus to ovarian follicular maturation[6]. In anorexia nervosa, LH secretion is often very low, and cyclical release may be absent, similar to the situation found in prepubertal children.

THE ROLE OF OPIATES AND DOPAMINE

A number of studies have attempted to evaluate the relevance of opiates and dopamine to hypothalamic amenorrhoea and weight-related amenorrhoea. The results have been conflicting. Yen and colleagues showed that both opiate and dopamine antagonists elicited significant increases in LH levels in patients with hypothalamic amenorrhoea, and that the opiate antagonist amplified the pulsatile pattern of LH release, suggesting a direct hypothalamic effect[7]. However, these effects were only seen in some women, and not in those with prepubertal levels of LH and a lower concentration of oestradiol. In other studies of hypo-oestrogenic women with weight-related amenorrhoea, opiate antagonists had no effect on LH pulsatility[8,9]. Blankstein and colleagues noted a strong U-shaped relationship between the ambient levels of circulatory oestradiol and the LH pulsatile responses to opiate antagonists[3]. This study included hyperprolactinaemic as well as normal women and the results are difficult to interpret for this reason. However, it is clear that responders to opiate antagonists had much higher levels of oestradiol than did non-responders. Thus, in some women with hypothalamic amenorrhoea, opioidergic inhibition of GnRH release does appear to be responsible for the decreased pulse frequency, but this effect is itself dependent on peripheral sex steroids and not just on central control mechanisms. In those women with similar decreased LH pulsatility but low oestradiol concentrations, opiates do not appear to account for the inhibition of intrinsic GnRH pulsatility. However, in some patients who have coexisting hyperprolactinaemia, opiate antagonist therapy has been shown to increase LH release acutely[8], although the results of a recent study contradict this earlier finding[10]. There is no good evidence for a long-term beneficial effect of dopamine agonists or antagonists on LH pulsatility in patients with hypothalamic amenorrhoea or anorexia nervosa.

HYPOTHALAMIC PITUITARY ADRENAL AXIS IN ANOREXIA NERVOSA AND DEPRESSION

Anorexia nervosa is a psychiatric condition, with some neuroendocrinological findings identical to those found in depression. In both conditions there is persistent hypercortisolaemia, with urinary free cortisol levels

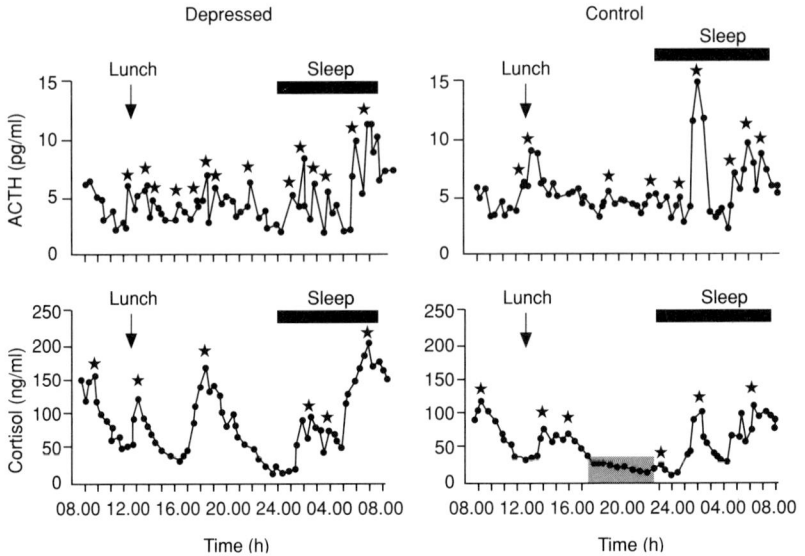

Figure 1 Diurnal rhythm of adrenocorticotrophin (ACTH) and cortisol in a patient with depression compared with a control subject. (From reference 13, with permission, © The Endocrine Society)

often in the range associated with Cushing's syndrome[11,12]. When studied in detail the diurnal rhythm of cortisol is preserved in these patients (in contrast to those with Cushing's syndrome), but there is a marked increase in episodic cortisol secretion and an increase in mean ACTH pulse frequency over 24 h compared to normal individuals, whereas the mean ACTH pulse amplitude and mean ACTH levels are similar to those in normal individuals[13] (Figure 1). These findings suggest that there is a centrally mediated activation of the hypothalamo–pituitary–adrenal axis. Interestingly, patients with depression and anorexia nervosa have a decreased ACTH response to CRF compared with controls, despite the presence of hypercortisolaemia, indicating an enhanced sensitivity of the adrenal gland to ACTH stimulation, but an appropriate corticotroph response to the excess adrenal glucocorticoid feedback[12,14], and whereas the adrenal response to ACTH returns to normal within 6 weeks of weight gain in patients with anorexia, a normal pituitary corticotroph response to CRF takes up to 6 months to become apparent. Other studies have shown that the level of both CRF and ACTH in the cerebrospinal fluid is much higher in depressed patients than in patients with Cushing's syndrome[15]. Indeed, CRF and ACTH levels in the CSF of patients with Cushing's syndrome are lower than in normal subjects, demonstrating not only that systemic ACTH does not cross the blood–brain barrier, but also that in Cushing's syndrome the increased production of corticosteroid does inhibit centrally produced CRF and ACTH. Since this does not occur in depression, it is likely that the increased pituitary–adrenocortical activity observed in this condition is due to an increased pulsatile release of intracerebral and/or hypothalamic release of CRF. This is of relevance to gonadal function since CRF has been shown to have powerful inhibitory effects on gonadotrophin release.

EFFECTS OF CRF ON GONADAL FUNCTION

Most of the work in this field has been performed in the rat and the conclusions have to be interpreted with caution when applied to the human or primate model since (unlike the rat) GnRH neuronal projections in the human extend outside the arcuate ventromedial nucleus of the hypothalamus[16]. However, the findings are of interest. Stress in the form of electric shock administered to recently castrated rats immediately and markedly decreases LH secretion and completely abolishes the pulsatility seen in these animals[17] (Figure 2). Central administration of CRF antiserum reverses this inhibitory effect, as does the intraventricular administration of a CRF antagonist. However, intravenous administration of the antagonist does not reverse the effects of stress, implying that CRF action is mediated centrally and is not affecting the pituitary release of GnRH. In another study assessing sexual activity in the rat, CRF infusion into the arcuate ventromedial area of the hypothalamus was associated with a prompt inhibition of lordosis behaviour[18]. Since CRF stimulates the release of β-endorphin as well as ACTH, the authors considered whether this effect was mediated by either of these peptides. Pretreatment of the rats with a specific β-endorphin antiserum prevented the inhibitory effects of CRF, but this was not found with an anti-ACTH antiserum. Indeed the effect was exaggerated with the latter. Concomitant intravenous administration of GnRH promptly reversed the inhibitory effects of CRF, indicating that the action was central.

A number of studies have now demonstrated that the inhibitory effect of CRF on GnRH release is at least in part opiate-mediated.

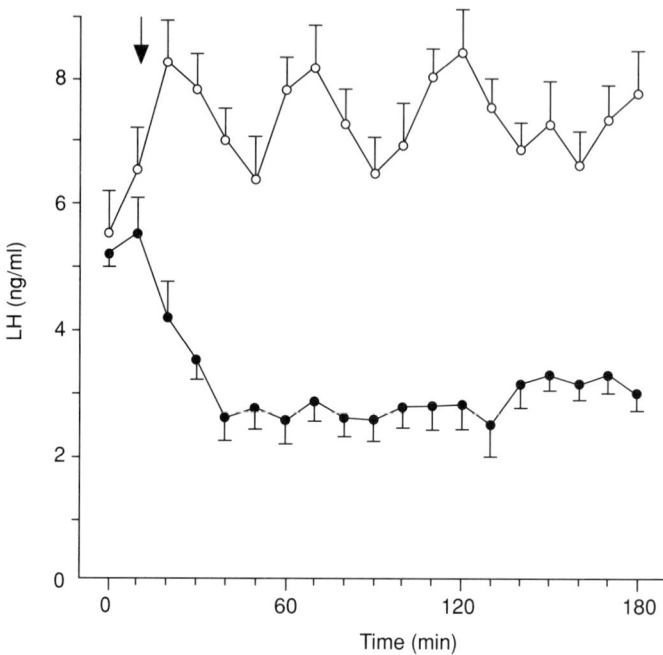

Figure 2 Effect of acute stress on luteinizing hormone (LH) secretion and pulsatility in recently castrated (•) male rats compared to control animals. Reproduced with permission from reference 17 (copyright 1986, AAAS)

More importantly, the effect of opiates can only be demonstrated in sex-primed or recently castrated animals in whom the central effects of sex steroids are still operative[19]. In long-term castrated animals, opiate antagonists have no effect on the CRF-induced fall in LH, which still occurs but is less marked than that in steroid-primed animals[20,21]. When CRF is injected into the mesencephalic grey area (also an important centre for control of sexual function in the rat), which contains β-endorphin- and ACTH-immunoreactive fibres, lordosis is inhibited, but pretreatment with an anti-β-endorphin antiserum at this site does not reverse the effect[18]. It thus seems likely that CRF inhibits GnRH release by at least two mechanisms, one of which involves opiates, and depends on the presence of endogenous sex steroids to mediate the inhibitory effect, and one which does not involve opiates. These observations would fit in very well with the divergent findings in women with hypothalamic amenorrhoea or anorexia given opiate antagonists.

In response to prolonged stress or anorexia nervosa, hypercortisolaemia may also be important due to its separate direct suppressive action on the pituitary release of gonadotrophins, since in Cushing's syndrome the gonadotroph response to GnRH is markedly attenuated, but is restored once the hypercortisolaemia is abolished[22]. Thus, in anorexia nervosa, changes in LH secretion could be explained by a non-opiate-mediated inhibitory effect of CRF on hypothalamic GnRH pulse frequency and corticosteroid-induced inhibition of pituitary gonadotrophin release causing decreased pulse amplitude.

OTHER EFFECTS OF STRESS ON PITUITARY HORMONE SECRETION

Electroshock therapy to rats is associated with a prompt inhibition of growth hormone release, which can be reversed by a CRF antagonist. CRF also directly inhibits basal and stimulated growth hormone secretion, but this can be reversed by concomitant administration of anti-somatostatin antiserum. Overall, the data suggest that CRF stimulates the secretion of somatostatin which is the direct inhibitor of both growth hormone releasing factor and growth hormone release[23].

Although hyperprolactinaemia is found in acute stressed states, it is not a feature of chronic anxiety or depression and is therefore unlikely to be relevant to the changes in LH pulsatility found in hypothalamic amenorrhoea or anorexia nervosa[24].

CONCLUSIONS

Normal, cyclical GnRH pulse frequency and amplitude is reduced in women with anorexia nervosa and hypothalamic amenorrhoea, and it is likely that higher cortical function has a major influence on this. The exact mechanisms responsible have to remain speculative, but on the basis of animal studies, an increase in intracerebral CRF (an acute and chronic stress peptide) causing inhibition of GnRH release, either directly or indirectly through an opioidergic pathway, has to be considered, and in anorexia nervosa, at least, increased central CRF activity has been demonstrated conclusively. While opiate antagonist therapy has been used to induce ovulation in some women with hypothalamic amenorrhoea[25], psychological counselling should also be considered for the treatment of this condition, just as it is used in anorexia nervosa. Finally, there are several other known factors which have inhibitory or stimulatory effects on the GnRH pulse generator and further studies are needed to ascertain their relevance to the changes in gonadotrophin secretion seen in hypothalamic amenorrhoea and anorexia nervosa.

REFERENCES

1. Ronkainen, H., Pakarinnen, A., Kirkinen, P. and Kauppila, A. (1985). Physical exercise-induced changes and season-associated differences in the pituitary-ovarian function of runners and joggers. *J. Clin. Endocrinol. Metab.*, **60**, 416–22

2. Quigley, M. E. and Yen, S. S. C. (1980). Role of endogenous opiates on LH secretion during the menstrual cycle. *J. Clin. Endocrinol. Metab.*, **51**, 179–81

3. Blankstein, J., Reyes, F. I., Winter, J. S. D. and Faiman, C. (1981). Endorphins and the regulation of human menstrual cycle. *Clin. Endocrinol.*, **14**, 287–94

4. Quigley, M. E., Judd, S. J., Gilliland, G. B. and Yen, S. S. C. (1979). Effects of a dopamine antagonist on the release of gonadotrophin and prolactin in normal women with hyperprolactinaemic anovulation. *J. Clin. Endocrinol. Metab.*, **48**, 718–20

5. Zumoff, B., Freeman, R., Couper, S., Saenger, P., Markowitz, M. and Kresna, J. (1983). A chronobiological abnormality in luteinizing hormone secretion in teenage girls with the polycystic ovary syndrome. *N. Engl. J. Med.*, **309**, 1206–9

6. Reame, N. E., Sauder, S. E., Case, G. D., Kelch, R. P. and Marshall, J. C. (1985). Pulsatile gonadotrophin secretion in women with hypothalamic amenorrhoea: Evidence that reduced frequency of gonadotrophin releasing hormone secretion is the mechanism of persistent anovulation. *J. Clin. Endocrinol. Metab.*, **61**, 851–8

7. Quigley, M. E., Sheehan, K. L., Casper, R. F. and Yen, S. S. C. (1980). Evidence for increased dopaminergic and opioid activity in patients with hypothalamic hypogonadotrophic amenorrhoea. *J. Clin. Endocrinol. Metab.*, **50**, 949–54

8. Grossman, A., Moult, P. J. A., McIntyre, H., Evans, J., Silverstone, T., Rees,

L.H. and Besser, G.M. (1982). Opiate mediation of amenorrhoea in hyperprolactinaemia and in weight loss related amenorrhea. *Clin. Endocrinol.*, **17**, 379–88

9. Armeanu, M.C., Berkhout, G.M.J. and Shoemaker, J. (1992). Pulsatile luteinizing hormone secretion in hypothalamic amenorrhoea, anorexia, and polycystic ovarian disease during naltrexone treatment. *Fertil. Steril.*, **57**, 762–70

10. Tay, C.C.K., Glasier, A.F., Illingworth, P.J. and Baird, D.T. (1993). Abnormal twenty-four pattern of pulsatile luteinizing hormone secretion and the response to naxolone in women with hyperprolactinaemic amenorrhoea. *Clin. Endocrinol.*, **39**, 599–606

11. Boyar, R.M., Hellman, L.D., Roffwarg, H., Katz, J., Zumoff, B., O'Connor, J., Bradlow, H.L. and Fukushima, D.K. (1977). Cortisol secretion and metabolism in anorexia nervosa. *N. Engl. J. Med.*, **296**, 190–3

12. Gold, P.W., Loriaux, D.L., Roy, A., Kling, M.A., Calabrese, J.R., Kellner, C.H., Nieman, L.K., Post, R.M., Pickar, D., Gallucci, W., Avgerinus, P., Paul, S., Oldfield, E.H., Cutler, G.B. and Crousos, G.P. (1986). Responses to corticotrophin-releasing hormone in the hypercortisolism of depression and Cushing's disease. *N. Engl. J. Med.*, **314**, 1329–35

13. Mortola, J.F., Liu, J.H., Gillim, J.C., Rasmussen, D.D. and Yen, S.S.C. (1987). Pulsatile rhythms of adrenocorticotrophin (ACTH) and cortisol in women with endogenous depression: evidence for increased ACTH pulse frequency. *J. Clin. Endocrinol. Metab.*, **65**, 962–8

14. Gold, P.W., Gwietsman, H., Avgerinos, P.C., Nieman, L.K., Gallucci, W.T., Kaye, W., Jimerson, D., Ebert, M., Rittmaster, R., Loriaux, L. and Crousos, G.P. (1986). Abnormal hypothalamic-pituitary-adrenal function in anorexia nervosa. *N. Engl. J. Med.*, **314**, 1335–42

15. Kling, M.A., Roy, A., Dorn, A.R., Calabrese, J.R., Rubinow, D.R., Whitfield, H.J., May, C., Post, R.M., Crousos, G.P., and Gold, P.W. (1991). Cerebrospinal fluid immunoreactive corticotropin-releasing hormone and adrenocorticotropin secretion in Cushing's disease and major depression: potential clinical implications. *J. Clin. Endocrinol. Metab.*, **76**, 260–71

16. King, J.C. and Anthony, E.L.P. (1984). LHRH neurons and their projections in humans and other mammals: species comparisons. *Peptides*, **5** (suppl. 1), 195–207

17. Rivier, C., Rivier, J. and Vale, W. (1986). Stress-induced inhibition of reproductive functions: role of endogenous corticotropin-releasing factor. *Science*, **231**, 607–9

18. Sirinathsinghli, D.J.S., Rees, L.H., Rivier, J. and Vale, W. (1983). Corticotropin-releasing factor is a potent inhibitor of sexual receptivity in the female rat. *Nature (London)*, **305**, 232–5

19. Bhanot, R. and Wilkinson, M. (1983). Opiatergic control of LH secretion is eliminated by gonadectomy. *Endocrinology*, **112**, 399–400

20. Rivier, C. and Vale, W. (1984). Influence of corticotropin-releasing factor on reproductive functions in the rat. *Endocrinology*, **114**, 914–20

21. Almeida, O.F.X., Nikolarakis, K.E. and Herz, A. (1988). Evidence for the involvement of endogenous opioids in the inhibition of luteinizing hormone by corticotropin-releasing factor. *Endocrinology*, **122**, 1034–41

22. White, M.C., Sanderson, J., Mashiter, K. and Joplin, G.F. (1981). Serum gonadotrophin levels in women with Cushing's syndrome before and after treatment. *Clin. Endocrinol.*, **14**, 23–9

23. Rivier, C. and Vale, W. (1985). Involvement of corticotropin-releasing factor and somatostatin in stress-induced inhibition of growth hormone secretion in the rat. *Endocrinology*, **117**, 2478–82

24. Delitala, G., Tomasi, P. and Virdis, R. (1987). Hormone secretion during stress. *Clin. Endocrinol. Metab.*, **1**, 391–414

25. Wildt, T. and Leyendecker, G. (1987). Induction of ovulation by the chronic administration of naltrexone in hypothalamic amenorrhoea. *J. Clin. Endocrinol. Metab.*, **64**, 1334–41

6

Hypersecretion of luteinizing hormone in polycystic ovary syndrome: causes and consequences

S. Franks, D. M. White and D. W. Polson

INTRODUCTION

Although hypersecretion of luteinizing hormone (LH) in the face of normal serum follicle stimulating hormone (FSH) concentrations is a characteristic feature of the biochemistry of polycystic ovary syndrome (PCOS) [1,2], serum concentrations of LH are not invariably elevated in women with this condition. The purpose of this review is to discuss the factors which may influence tonic secretion of LH in women with polycystic ovaries. Elevated LH concentrations may, in turn, affect ovarian function; the role of LH in follicular maturation and the possible effects of high LH levels on fertility will be reviewed.

PREVALENCE OF ELEVATED SERUM LH LEVELS IN WOMEN WITH POLYCYSTIC OVARIES

The prevalence of raised serum concentrations of LH in any given series of patients with PCOS will depend on the criteria for the diagnosis of the condition. In other words, if hypersecretion of LH is taken as a *sine qua non* for the diagnosis, all patients will, by definition, have elevated LH concentrations. In a series of 300 women presenting to a single gynae-cological endocrine clinic with symptoms of hyperandrogenism or anovulation (or both), and in whom the primary criterion for the diagnosis of PCOS was the ultrasound morphology of the ovaries, 51% had a baseline LH concentration above the upper limit of the normal range [2,3]. Those women who presented with menstrual disturbance were more likely to have an elevated LH level (63%) than those with hirsutism who presented with regular cycles (21%). Nevertheless, the median LH concentration was significantly higher in hirsute women with regular cycles than in control subjects with normal ovaries [2,3].

Because of the episodic nature of LH secretion, random measurements of serum levels may not be a reliable guide to the underlying pattern of LH secretion. We therefore undertook a study in 33 anovulatory women with polycystic ovaries, taking blood samples at 15-min intervals for 8 h. Gonadotrophin measurements were compared with those in a control group of seven subjects with normal ovaries, sampled in the early to mid-follicular phase of an ovulatory, menstrual cycle. As expected, the 8-h mean LH concentrations and the amplitude of LH pulses were significantly higher in women with PCOS than in normal subjects (Table 1). There was, however, no overall increase in pulse frequency. Serial sampling of LH concentrations proved a more sensitive method of detecting hypersecretion of LH than random samples; 27 of 33 women with PCOS had an 8-h mean LH level above the upper limit of normal in the control group, whereas only 19 of the 33 women had a raised LH level on random sampling. Nevertheless, there was considerable heterogeneity between individuals in the pattern of LH secretion and, importantly, there remained six subjects (18%) whose 8-h mean LH level fell within the normal range. These women were, by definition, anovulatory and had polycystic ovaries. In addition, all had hirsutism and/or raised androgen levels.

The definition of elevated LH levels is also affected by the method used to assay LH in the circulation. There has been a recent plethora of immunoradiometric methods for LH assay, predominantly employing specific monoclonal antisera. The results obtained by such assays may not accord directly with those derived from the more traditional radioimmuno-assay using polyclonal antisera [4,5]. In general, although immunoradiometric assays may be more sensitive than radioimmunoassays, the latter are better than the former at detecting higher levels of LH and, importantly, values obtained by radioimmunoassay show a better correlation with levels of bioactive LH [5].

Table 1 Pulsatile luteinizing hormone (LH) secretion in anovulatory women with polycystic ovary syndrome (PCOS). Values are mean ± SD

Group	n	8-h mean LH (U/l)	Pulse amplitude (U/l)	Frequency (pulses/8 h)
Control	7	4.3 ± 1.3	1.7 ± 0.7	4.8 ± 1.2
PCOS				
total	33	13.1 ± 6.8★★†	5.3 ± 3.5★	6.0 ± 2.1
high basal LH	19	17.2 ± 5.7★★	6.5 ± 1.3★★	6.9 ± 3.1★

Significantly different from control: ★ $p < 0.05$; ★★ $p < 0.01$, Student's *t*-test on log-transformed data; † 6 of 33 (18%) of women with PCOS had an 8-h mean LH value which was < 6.9 U/l (i.e. < 2 SD above the mean of the control group)

MECHANISM OF INCREASED LH SECRETION IN PCOS

It has been suggested that abnormal LH secretion in women with PCOS results from primary dysregulation of gonadotrophin secretion by the hypothalamus[6]. This has been postulated on the basis of a higher than normal frequency of LH pulses and on the observation of abnormal diurnal gonadotrophin release in adolescent girls with clinical features of PCOS[6,7]. Not all studies have been able to demonstrate an overall increase in LH pulse frequency[2]. Again, much depends on the criteria for diagnosis of PCOS. In patients selected on the basis of elevated random LH values, both amplitude *and* frequency of LH pulses are greater than normal, whereas those women with normal random LH levels have higher than normal 24-h mean values and pulse amplitude but normal frequency. Increased pulse frequency could, in any event, be explained by abnormal steroid feedback at the hypothalamic level.

In a recent study of pituitary responsiveness to exogenous gonadotrophin releasing hormone (GnRH) in women with PCOS, we noted that women with anovulatory cycles have a greatly exaggerated response to a single dose of a GnRH agonist analogue compared with either normal subjects or ovulatory hyperandrogenaemic women with polycystic ovaries (Figure 1). These findings suggest that lack of the normal cyclical changes in ovarian steroids – in particular, progesterone deficiency – may be one of the most significant factors influencing tonic hypersecretion of LH.

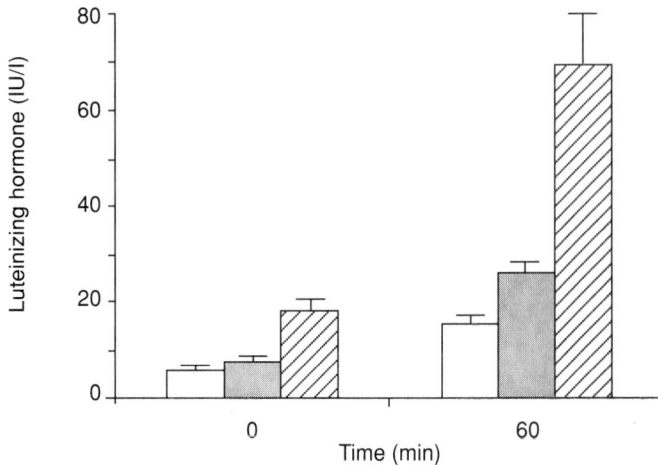

Figure 1 Luteinizing hormone (LH) response (mean ± SE) to a single dose (100 μg) of gonadotrophin releasing hormone analogue (buserelin) in controls (□), ovulatory women with polycystic ovaries (ovPCO; ▨) and anovulatory women with polycystic ovaries (anov PCO; ▨). The concentrations of LH at 60 min were significantly different from normal in both groups of PCO women but the levels in anovPCO were higher than in ovPCO. (ovPCO *vs.* control $p < 0.005$; anovPCO *vs.* control, $p < 0.001$; anovPCO *vs.* ovPCO, $p < 0.001$; Student's *t*-test)

This is further borne out by the significant suppression of LH concentrations seen during spontaneous or induced ovulatory cycles in anovulatory women with PCOS[2]. Nevertheless, examination of the pituitary response to GnRHa in *ovulatory* women with PCOS (Figure 1) reveals that even in these subjects there is a small, but significant, increase in LH secretion, compared with normal subjects. This is in keeping with previous findings reported on baseline LH measurements[2,3]. One hypothesis, which remains to be proven, is that secretion of LH in women with PCOS represents conditioning or 'masculinization' of the pituitary in response to excessive androgen levels during development[8,9]. This suggestion is supported by the finding of an exaggerated LH response in the initial stage of stimulation by GnRH agonist analogues, a pattern which is characteristic of that in men[8,9]. Furthermore, it has been shown that patients with a history of neonatal exposure to hyperandrogenaemia as a result of 21–hydroxylase deficency, also show an enhanced LH response to GnRH agonist analogues in later life[10].

CONSEQUENCES OF ELEVATED LH CONCENTRATIONS IN WOMEN WITH PCOS

Conway and colleagues, in an analysis of over 500 women with polycystic ovaries, reported that hypersecretion of LH was associated with subfertility[11]. The association between elevated LH levels and subfertility is also apparent in women who undergo superovulation or induction of ovulation. Data from *in vitro* fertilization programmes have shown that inappropriately elevated serum LH concentrations during the phase of follicular stimulation are associated with low rates of fertilization and of successful pregnancy[12,13].

An adverse effect of raised serum LH concentrations on fertility and miscarriage in spontaneous or induced ovulatory cycles has also been reported[14–17]. In our studies of women treated with low–dose gonadotrophins, elevated pretreatment levels of LH (which occurred in 53% of patients treated) were associated with a lower rate of ovulation than that in subjects with normal baseline LH levels[17]. However, the more important predictor of outcome of treatment was the mid-follicular phase concentration of LH. Serum LH concentrations tend to fall towards the normal range during treatment with either follicle stimulating hormone or human menopausal gonadotrophin but in some 25% of ovulatory cycles, LH concentrations remain higher than normal. This appears to have an adverse effect on outcome. In only one of 12 such cycles did successful pregnancy occur, compared with 54% of cycles in which the mid-follicular phase LH concentration was normal[17].

These data raise the question of whether suppression of LH during induction of ovulation would improve the successful pregnancy rate. Results from the few randomized studies that have compared the effects of gonadotrophin treatment, with or without GnRH agonist analogues, remain unconvincing[18].

The above discussion draws attention to the association between raised LH levels and subfertility and/or miscarriage, without establishing cause and effect. However, *in vitro* studies of LH action on preovulatory follicles suggest a mechanism by which elevated LH levels may have a direct adverse effect on the outcome of treatment. In the later stages of development of the dominant follicle, granulosa cells possess functional LH receptors. LH has been shown to have a dose-related stimulatory effect on steroidogenesis but, at the same time, inhibits granulosa cell proliferation in a dose-dependent fashion[19]. This would account for the inhibition of granulosa cell mitosis which occurs, physiologically, at the start of the LH surge, but may also explain why patients with polycystic ovaries who have elevated levels of LH may fail to develop a pre-ovulatory follicle. In other words, if the maturing follicle is exposed to supraphysiological levels of LH before the onset of the surge, maturation 'arrest' may occur.

SUMMARY

Hypersecretion of LH in women with PCOS can be explained on the basis of 'conditioning' of the pituitary response to GnRH by androgens. This effect may be considerably exaggerated by lack of the normal cyclical feedback pattern in anovulatory subjects with PCOS. Hypersecretion of LH may, in turn, have an adverse effect on the developing follicle by contributing to the premature maturation arrest of granulosa cells.

REFERENCES

1. Yen, S.C.C. (1980). The polycystic ovary syndrome. *Clin. Endocrinol.*, **12**, 177–207
2. Franks, S. (1989). Polycystic ovary syndrome: a changing perspective. *Clin. Endocrinol.*, **31**, 87–120
3. Adams, J., Polson, D.W. and Franks, S. (1986). Prevalence of polycystic ovaries in women with anovulation and idiopathic hirsutism. *Br. Med. J.*, **293**, 355–9
4. Fauser, B.C., Pache, T.D., Lamberts, S.W., Hop, W.C., de Jong, F. and Dahl, K.D. (1991). Serum bioactive and immunoreactive luteinizing hormone and follicle-stimulating hormone levels in women with cycle abnormalities, with or without polycystic ovarian disease. *J. Clin. Endocrinol. Metab.*, **73**, 811–17
5. Fauser, B.C., Pache, T.D., Hop, W.C., de Jong, F. and Dahl, K.D. (1992). The significance of a single serum LH measurement in women with cycle disturbances: discrepancies between immunoreactive and bioactive hormone estimates. *Clin. Endocrinol.*, **37**, 445–52

6. Waldstreicher, J., Santoro, N. F., Hall, J. E., Filicori, M. and Crowley, W. J. (1988). Hyperfunction of the hypothalamic-pituitary axis in women with polycystic ovarian disease: indirect evidence for partial gonadotrope desensitization. *J. Clin. Endocrinol. Metab.*, **66**, 165–72

7. Zumoff, B., Freeman, R., Coupey, S., Saenger, P., Markowitz, M. and Kream, J. (1983). A chronobiologic abnormality of luteinizing hormone secretion in teenage girls with the polycystic ovary syndrome. *N. Engl. J. Med.*, **309**, 1206–9

8. Barnes, R. B., Rosenfield, R. L., Burstein, S. and Ehrmann, D. A. (1989). Pituitary–ovarian responses to nafarelin testing in the polycystic ovary syndrome. *N. Engl. J. Med.*, **320**, 559–65

9. Rosenfield, R. L., Barnes, R. B., Cara, J. F. and Lucky, A. W. (1990). Dysregulation of cytochrome P450c 17 alpha as the cause of polycystic ovarian syndrome. *Fertil. Steril.*, **53**, 785–91

10. Barnes, R. B., Ehrmann, D. A. and Rosenfield, R. L. (1993). Ovarian hyper-androgenism in 'late-onset' congenital adrenal hyperplasia. *Proceedings of the Endocrine Society 75th Annual Meeting*, abstract 128 (The Endocrine Society)

11. Conway, G. S., Honour, J. W. and Jacobs, H. S.(1989). Heterogeneity of the polycystic ovary syndrome: clinical, endocrine and ultrasound features in 556 patients. *Clin. Endocrinol.*, **30**, 459–70

12. Stanger, J. D. and Yovich, J. L. (1985). Reduced *in vitro* fertilisation of human oocytes from patients with raised basal luteinising hormone levels during the follicular phase. *Br. J. Obstet. Gynaecol.*, **92**, 385–90

13. Howles, C. M., MacNamee, M. C., Edwards, R. G., Goswamy, R. and Steptoe, P. C. (1986). Effect of high tonic levels of luteinising hormone on outcome of *in vitro* fertilisation. *Lancet*, **2**, 521–3

14. Regan, L., Owen, E. J. and Jacobs, H. S., (1990). Hypersecretion of luteinising hormone, infertility and miscarriage. *Lancet*, **336**, 1141–4

15. Watson, H., Kiddy, D. S., Hamilton-Fairley, D., Scanlon, M. J., Barnard, C., Collins, W. P., Bonney, R. and Franks, S., (1993). Hypersecretion of luteinizing hormone and ovarian steroids in women with recurrent early miscarriage. *Hum. Reprod.*, **8**, 829–33

16. Homburg, R., Armar, N. A., Eshel, A., Adams, J. and Jacobs H. S. (1988). Influence of serum luteinising hormone concentrations on ovulation, conception and early pregnancy loss in polycystic ovary syndrome. *Br. Med. J.*, **297**, 1024–6

17. Hamilton-Fairley, D., Kiddy, D., Watson, H., Sagle, M. and Franks, S. (1991). Low-dose gonadotrophin therapy for induction of ovulation in 100 women with polycystic ovary syndrome. *Hum. Reprod.*, **6**, 1095–9

18. Schoot, D. C., Pijlman, B., Stijnen, T. and Fauser, B. C., (1992). Effects of gonadotrophin releasing hormone agonist addition to gonatotrophin

induction of ovulation in polycystic ovary syndrome patients. *Eur. J. Obstet. Gynecol. Reprod Biol.*, **45**, 53–8

19. Yong, E.L., Baird, D.T., and Hillier, S.G. (1992). Mediation of gonadotrophin–stimulated growth and differentiation by human granulosa cells by adenosine-3',5'-monophosphate: one molecule, two messages. *Clin. Endocrinol.*, **37**, 51–8

7

Disorders of the thyroid and adrenal glands: effects on ovulation and pregnancy

M. de Swiet

THE THYROID GLAND

It is well-known that both hypo- and hyperthyroidism may cause abnormal ovulation. Indeed thyroid function should be assessed bio-chemically in all infertile women. Not infrequently such patients are found to be hypothyroid, or occasionally hyperthyroid, with no clinical evidence of the abnormality, and treatment of the thyroid disorder restores ovulation and fertility.

Hypothyroidism

The mechanism(s) by which hypo- and hyperthyroidism cause ovulatory failure are not clear. Hypothyroidism has been associated with progesterone excess[1] leading to endometrial proliferation. A more obvious cause of ovulatory failure is prolactin excess. Patients with hypothyroidism have high levels of thyrotropin releasing hormone (TRH) because of loss of the negative feedback of thyroxine on TRH release. TRH, besides stimu-lating release of thyroid stimulating hormone (TSH) from the anterior pituitary, also allows prolactin release. However, this cannot be the sole mechanism by which low thyroxine levels are associated with ovulatory failure since some patients have normal prolactin levels. Furthermore some patients have achieved pregnancy despite gross hypothyroidism[2].

It has been reported that pregnancy failure is more common in hypo-thyroid patients for a variety of reasons, including preterm labour and accidental haemorrhage[3]. In practice this is likely to be an excessively pessimistic view: once hypothyroid women become pregnant, their pregnancies seem to be no more complicated than those of normal women.

Whether doses of thyroxine replacement need to be increased in pregnancy is disputed. Mandel and co-workers[4] monitored free thyroxine and TSH levels, and found that nine of 12 patients needed an increase in thyroxine dose from about 100 μg/day before pregnancy to about 150 μg/day during pregnancy. In a larger series of 25 patients, we found that such dosage adjustments were not necessary if the TSH level at the beginning of pregnancy indicated adequate replacement[5].

Hyperthyroidism

Although hyperthyroidism tends to remit in pregnancy, its management is a greater cause for concern than is the management of hypothyroidism. This is because of the possible effects in the foetus of maternal therapy and the transplacental passage of thyroid-stimulating antibodies.

Treatment options are antithyroid drugs and surgery. Radioiodine is used with reluctance in young women and should never be used in pregnancy since it will also ablate the foetal thyroid. Surgery is usually reserved for those patients with evidence of obstruction, those who fail to respond to medical therapy, and those who are unlikely to be able to comply with medical therapy for personal or social reasons.

In the UK, commonly used antithyroid drugs are propylthiouracil (PTU) and carbimazole. Although there is less experience in general with the use of PTU than with carbimazole, it is probably the agent of choice for pregnancy: it decreases thyroid stimulating immunoglobulin (TSI) levels independently of reducing thyroxine synthesis; it is less likely to cause malformations such as aplasia cutis in the foetus[6] and less is secreted in breast milk[7,8]. Antithyroid drugs are one of the very few classes of drugs that can be secreted in breast milk in amounts sufficient to harm the infant[9]. The principle of antithyroid treatment in pregnancy is to give the minimum dose of antithyroid drug required to control maternal free thyroxine levels. The foetus should then not be affected. There seems to be no place for a combination of maximal antithyroid drug treatment supported by thyroxine, a regimen which has been advocated in the past[10,11]. Antithyroid drugs do cross the placenta and high doses could easily render the foetus hypothyroid[12,13]. Since relatively little thyroxine crosses the placenta, even if the mother is protected from excessive thyroid inhibition, the foetus would not be.

Neonatal hyperthyroidism

Neonatal hyperthyroidism caused by maternal TSI crossing the placenta is an important and perplexing problem. It occurs in up to 10% of neonates whose mothers had Graves' disease in pregnancy[1]. Maternal TSI levels > 20 units/ml are accurate in predicting neonatal hyperthyroidism[14] but unfortunately this assay is not widely available and in any case the baby is usually delivered by the time that the results are known.

Hyperthyroidism may be expressed *in utero*: the affected foetus becomes growth-retarded or delivery is difficult because of goitre[15,16]; both of these manifestations are very rare. The condition may be obvious at birth, or its appearance may be delayed until the second week of life. It is clear that some other factor or factors modulate the clinical manifestation of neonatal hyperthyroidism: this has tentatively been ascribed to 'blocking' antibodies[17,18]. This is similar to the inhibition of the expression of motor end-plate antibodies in foetuses carried by women with myasthenia gravis: the foetus is not affected *in utero* and only shows signs of neonatal myasthenia a few days after delivery.

The late appearance of neonatal hyperthyroidism is an important cause of the significant mortality associated with the condition. The infants have been discharged from hospital when they present and are no longer under routine paediatric surveillance. Infants born to all women who have had Graves' disease in pregnancy should be followed by a paediatrician for at least the first month of their lives.

Postpartum autoimmune thyroiditis

Late presentation is also the reason why transient postpartum autoimmune thyroiditis can be devastating. This condition is surprisingly common and occurs in at least 10% of Welsh and Japanese women. Affected women usually have evidence of pre-existing thyroid disease as indicated by thyroid microsomal autoantibodies. Between 3 and 6 months after delivery their autoimmune disease flares, usually with cytotoxic activity. They have a brief episode of hyperthyroxinaemia when the thyroid cells are destroyed followed by a longer, reversible period of hypothyroidism. These patients have been discharged from hospital care and there is an insufficient knowledge of the condition in the community. Their symptoms of depression and exhaustion are ascribed to motherhood, and they are reassured that they will get better spontaneously. Although this is so, many months of misery could be alleviated by a relatively short course of thyroxine treatment.

THE ADRENAL GLAND

Addison's disease

Patients with Addison's disease do not ovulate. This may be due to their general debilitation or more specifically because of loss of weight, i.e. they fail to achieve the critical weight necessary for ovulation that has been demonstrated in athletes and women with anorexia nervosa. An even more specific mechanism would be related to elevated levels of corticotrophin releasing factor (CRF). Direct intracerebral injection of CRF into rats inhibits gonadotrophin release and ovulation and interrupts pregnancy[19,20]. In primates, intravenous injection of CRF lowers gonadotrophin levels[21]. Excessive production of CRF may be the mechanism whereby 'stress' inhibits ovulation in humans (see Chapter 5).

Cushing's syndrome

Patients with Cushing's syndrome also have menstrual irregularity and may fail to ovulate. This may be due to the general effect of excessive androgen activity or may specifically relate to excessive glucocorticoid activity.

Congenital adrenal hyperplasia

Congenital adrenal hyperplasia (CAH) is a generic term applied to at least seven different rare abnormalities of adrenal steroidogenesis associated with hyperplasia of the adrenal glands[22]. Of these, 21-hydroxylase deficiency is by far the most common, accounting for about 95%

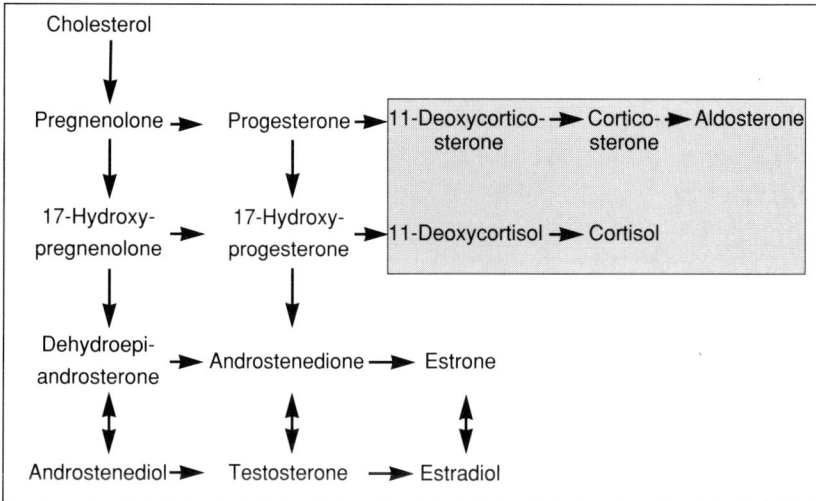

Figure 1 Pathways of adrenal steroid biosynthesis. The shaded area indicates steroids whose synthesis is impaired by a defect in secretion of the enzyme 21-hydroxylase, particularly cortisol and aldosterone. 21-Hydroxylase deficiency also causes the accumulation of the precursor 17-hydroxyprogesterone which leads to increased secretion of androstenedione and testosterone. (Reproduced with permission from ref. 33)

of cases of CAH. The metabolic defects are shown in Figure 1. In essence, the absence of 21-hydroxylase stops the conversion of progesterone to corticosterone and aldosterone and conversion of 17-hydroxyprogesterone to cortisol. The reduction in glucocorticoid and mineralocorticoid levels leads to excessive CRF and adrenocorticotrophin (ACTH) levels. ACTH increases adrenal biosynthesis and substances synthesized before the metabolic block accumulate, specifically 17-hydroxyprogesterone (17-OHP), which is used as a diagnostic and therapeutic marker, and androstenedione, which can be converted to testosterone and which itself has weak androgenic effects.

Anovulation in CAH

Inhibition of ovulation might be due to the excess of androgens or more specifically to elevated CRF levels (see above). Certainly, glucocorticoid treatment that suppresses ACTH, as shown by normal 17-OHP levels, is more likely to be associated with a normal menstrual pattern. However, both excess androgen and high CRF levels would be reduced by such treatment. Many patients with CAH also have polycystic ovaries, though it is not clear whether this causes or is an effect of high androgen levels. The separation of ovarian from adrenal causes of excess androgen activity, including mild late-onset adrenal hyperplasia due to 21-hydroxylase deficiency[23], is a major challenge[24] and beyond the scope of this paper.

21-Hydroxylase deficiency may be subdivided into the simple virilizing type, the more severe salt-losing variety and the mild late-onset variety referred to above. These differences must relate to heterogeneity in the complex gene differences that are currently being evaluated[22,25]. However, it is quite clear that the failure of women affected by virilizing and salt-losing forms of CAH to become pregnant relates to many more problems than simple failure to ovulate. Surgical procedures may be necessary to reduce the size of the clitoris, to divert the urinary stream away from the clitoris and to provide an adequate vagina for sexual intercourse. Such procedures have a major impact on the psychological adjustment of these women to femininity. In addition, perception of herself as female may have been altered by androgenic influences on the developing brain, both *in utero* and as a child.

Reproductive disorders in CAH

Mulaikal and colleagues[26] studied 80 females with 21-hydroxylase deficiency of the virilizing and salt-losing forms. The sexual behaviour of these patients was also compared to normal females[27], using Kinsey's statistics[28]. The results were not encouraging (Table 1). For example, only 55% of the patients with simple virilizing CAH had normal menstruation, despite the fact that they were treated in a centre of excellence. Only 60% were heterosexually active and only 60% had achieved successful pregnancy. Mulaikal and colleagues[26] correlated sexual activity with the adequacy of the introitus, but Federman[27] comments that the patient's perception of her introitus will very much depend on gender imprinting in early life and that this may also be a major problem. The brain of a male finch, for example, has a different shape from that of the female finch, and it sings differently[29]; these differences are androgen-dependent. Money and co-workers[30] noted a relatively high incidence of bisexuality and homosexuality in females with CAH, and they ascribed this to intra-uterine exposure to androgen.

Table 1 Menstrual function, marital status, sexual behaviour, and fertility in 80 adults with congenital adrenal hyperplasia and in normal adults. Data are given as percentages. (From ref. 27, with permission)

	Normal adults	Congenital adrenal hyperplasia	
		Simple	*Salt-losing*
Normal menses	87	55	67
Married (ever)	90	50	12.5
Introitus adequate	98	83	48
Heterosexually active	75–90	60	37
No sexual experience	~ 5	30	60
Fertility ratio	~90	60	2.5

Prevention of CAH

It is not surprising that major efforts are being made to normalize the intrauterine endocrine environment of foetuses at risk of CAH. The obvious strategy is to give the mother a glucocorticoid such as dexamethasone which freely crosses the placenta (in contrast to prednisone) and which could inhibit excessive ACTH production by the foetus *in utero*. Early attempts used such treatment in the second trimester, after it had been established that the foetus was female, and after amniotic fluid hormone analysis and HLA typing indicated that it was likely to be affected. However, although suppression of the foetal adrenals was demonstrated by a reduction in maternal serum oestriol, the foetuses were still virilized. It is now realized that gender differentiation occurs as early as 9 weeks after conception; such treatment should therefore start before this time, and preferably before 7 weeks of gestation. In practice this means treatment initially in all at-risk pregnancies, although treatment can be withheld if the foetus is found to be male or proved not to have CAH on the basis of genetic studies performed on material obtained by chorionic villus sampling.

Even treatment early in the first trimester prevents virilization in only about one-third of foetuses with CAH[31]. Another one-third of the infants show less severe degrees of virilization, and the remaining one-third are not affected by therapy. Other as yet unknown genetic or environmental factors must, therefore, also be involved[32]. Nevertheless, it is still worth pursuing such treatment, even if only two-thirds of the patients are helped. Multicentre studies may provide the clues to success in the remaining one-third of patients.

Pregnancy and CAH

In the cases considered above, it is usually not the mother but the foetus that has CAH. If the mother has CAH there is a small chance that her foetus will have CAH, depending on her partner's genotype. The *a priori* chance that he will be a carrier for some form of CAH can be reduced by genetic linkage studies, depending on the number of mutations that are looked for.

The pregnant woman with CAH needs continuing glucocorticoid therapy, preferably with prednisone or hydrocortisone, since these do not cross the placenta. The dose does not usually vary much from that administered before pregnancy, but it must be adjusted on the basis of clinical criteria, since 17-OHP levels increase in a variable manner due to pregnancy itself. In our limited experience such patients have a high incidence of pre-eclampsia and eclampsia. Caesarean section is often necessary because affected women have an android pelvis, again the result of androgen excess in early life.

REFERENCES

1. Ramsey, I. (1994). Thyroid disease. In de Swiet, M. (ed.) *Medical Disorders in Obstetric Practice*, 3rd edn. (Oxford: Blackwell Scientific Publications), in press
2. Balen, A.H. and Kurtz, A.B. (1990). Successful outcome of pregnancy with severe hypothyroidism. Case report and literature review. *Br. J. Obstet. Gynaecol.*, **97**, 536–9
3. Niswander, K.R. and Gordon, M. (1972). *The Women and Their Pregnancies.* (Philadelphia: W.B. Saunders)
4. Mandel, S.J., Larsen, P.R., Seely, E.W. and Brent, G.A. (1990). Increased need for thyroxine during pregnancy in women with primary hypo-thyroidism. *N. Engl. J. Med.*, **323**, 91–6
5. Girling, J.C. and de Swiet, M. (1992). Thyroxine dosage during pregnancy in women with primary hypothyroidism. *Br. J. Obstet. Gynaecol.*, **99**, 368–70

6. Milham, S. Jr (1985). Scalp defects in infants of mothers treated for hyper-thyroidism with methimazole or carbimazole during pregnancy. *Teratology*, **32**, 321

7. Kampmann, J.P., Johansen, K., Hansen, J.M. and Helweg, J. (1980). Propylthiouracil in human milk: revision of dogma, *Lancet*, **1**, 736–8

8. Low, L.C.K., Lang, J. and Alexander, W.D. (1979). Excretion of carbi-mazole and propylthiouracil in breast milk. *Lancet*, **2**, 1011

9. Williams, R.H., Kay, G.A. and Jandorf, B.J. (1944). Thiouracil. Its absorption, distribution and excretion. *J. Clin. Invest.*, **23**, 613–27

10. Fraser, R. and Wilkinson, M. (1953). Simplified method of drug treatment for thyrotoxicosis using a uniform dosage of methyl thiouracil and added thyroxine. *Br. Med. J.*, **1**, 481–4

11. Selenkow, H.A., Birnbaum, M.D. and Hollander, C.S. (1973). Thyroid function and dysfunction during pregnancy. *Clin. Obstet. Gynecol.*, **16**, 66–108

12. Hamburger, J.L. (1972). Management of the pregnant hyperthyroid. *Obstet. Gynecol.*, **40**, 114–17

13. Mestman, J.H. (1985). Thyroid disease in pregnancy. *Clin. Perinatol.*, **12**, 651–67

14. Dirmikis, S.M. and Munro, D.S. (1975). Placental transmission of thyroid-stimulating immunoglobulins. *Br. Med. J.*, **2**, 665–6

15. Cove, D.H. and Johnston, P. (1985). Fetal hyperthyroidism: experience of treatment in four siblings. *Lancet*, **1**, 430–2

16. Daneman, D. and Howard, N.J. (1980). Neonatal thyrotoxicosis: intellectual impairment and craniosynostosis in later years. *J. Pediatr.*, **97**, 257–9

17. Zakarija, M., McKenzie, J.M. and Munro, D.S. (1983). Immunoglobulin G inhibitor of thyroid-stimulating antibody is a cause of delay in the onset of neonatal Graves' disease. *J. Clin. Invest.*, **72**, 1352–6

18. Zakarija, M., McKenzie, J.M. and Hoffman, W.H. (1986). Prediction and therapy of intrauterine and late-onset neonatal hyperthyroidism. *J. Clin. Endocrinol. Metab.*, **62**, 368–71

19. Rivier, C. and Vale, W. (1984). Influence of corticotropin-releasing factor on reproductive functions in the rat. *Endocrinology*, **114**, 914–21

20. Ono, N., Lumpkin, M.D., Sampson, W.K., McDonald, J.K. and McCann, S.M. (1984). Intrahypothalamic action of corticotropin-releasing factor (CRF) to inhibit growth hormone and LH release in the rat. *Life Sci.*, **35**, 1117–23

21. Olster, D.H. and Ferin, M. (1987). Corticotropin-releasing hormone inhibits gonadotropin secretion in the ovariectomized Rhesus monkey. *J. Clin. Endocrinol. Metab.*, **65**, 262–7

22. White, P.C., New, M.I. and Dupont, B. (1987). Congenital adrenal hyperplasia. *N. Engl. J. Med.*, **316**, 1580–6

23. Eldar-Geva, T., Hurwitz, A., Vecsei, P., Palti, Z., Mildwidsky, A. and Rosler, A. (1990). Secondary biosynthetic defects in women with late onset congenital adrenal hyperplasia. *N. Engl. J. Med.*, **323**, 855–63

24. Ehrmann, D.A., Rosenfield, R.L., Barnes, R.B., Brigell, D.F. and Sheikh, Z. (1992). Detection of functional ovarian hyperandrogenism in women with androgen excess. *N. Engl. J. Med.*, **327**, 157–62

25. Editorial. (1987). Congenital adrenal hyperplasia. *Lancet*, **2**, 663–4

26. Mulaikal, R.M., Migeon, C.J. and Jock, J.A. (1987). Fertility rates in female patients with congenital adrenal hyperplasia due to 21-hydroxylase deficiency. *N. Engl. J. Med.*, **316**, 178–82

27. Federman, D.D. (1987). Psychosexual adjustment in congenital adrenal hyperplasia. *N. Engl. J. Med.*, **316**, 209–11

28. Kinsey, A.C., Pomeroy, W.B., Martin, C.E. and Gebard, P.H. (1953). *Sexual Behaviour in the Human Female*. (Philadelphia: W.B. Saunders)

29. Nottebohm, F. and Arnold, A.P. (1976). Sexual dimorphism in vocal control area of the songbird brain. *Science*, **194**, 211–13

30. Money, J., Schwartz, M. and Lewis, V.G. (1984). Adult erotosexual status and fetal hormonal masculinisation and demasculinisation: 46, XX congenital virilizing adrenal hyperplasia and 46, XY androgen-insensitivity syndrome compared. *Psychoneuroendocrinology*, **9**, 405–14

31. Pang, S., Pollack, M.S., Marshall, R.N. and Immken, L. (1990). Prenatal treatment of congenital adrenal hyperplasia due to 21-hydroxylase deficiency. *N. Engl. J. Med.*, **322**, 111–15

32. Editorial. (1990). Prenatal treatment of congenital adrenal hyperplasia. *Lancet*, **335**, 510–11

33. Cutler, G.B. and Laue, L. (1990). Congenital adrenal hyperplasia due to 21-hydroxylase deficiency. *N. Engl. J. Med.*, **323**, 1806–13

8

Premature ovarian failure

I. D. Cooke

INTRODUCTION

Premature ovarian failure is one extreme of a normal event, the loss of oocytes, and may be described as occurring before the age of 40 years. Although some causes, such as chemotherapy, radiotherapy and surgery, are iatrogenic and other cases are associated with autoimmune disease which may be polyglandular, a considerable proportion of cases remains idiopathic. The condition is probably better termed hypergonadotrophic hypogonadism, as pregnancies do occur following the diagnosis which needs to be distinguished from a resistant ovary syndrome.

The mechanisms involved in the development of hypergonado-trophic hypogonadism are not clear but may involve abnormalities in follicle stimulating hormone (FSH) production, in the FSH receptor and in signal transduction to the two second-messenger systems. Systematic investigation is needed to distinguish hypergonadotrophic hypogonadism from resistant ovary syndrome, but which patients will subsequently remit, ovulate and become pregnant cannot yet be predicted. Treatments offered have included steroid replacement, down-regulation with gonadotrophin stimulation and steroids for autoimmune abnormalities. Probably of greater importance is the use of oocyte donation for these patients. The long-term problems of reduced bone mass and increased cardiovascular disease should be prevented by hormone replacement therapy.

Recent karotypic analyses show Xp and Xq deletions, particularly in women with amenorrhoea, but there may be mutations in the gene for the FSH receptor and luteinizing hormone (LH) β-gene DNA sequence differences have been found. Oocyte donation has changed the fertility perspective but raised important philosophical issues. Multiple embryo transfer at oocyte donation yields delivery rates in excess of 25%, changing the fertility perspective for these young women.

Many issues remain. Is premature ovarian failure only gross or is it also a mild elevation in plasma FSH, failure to respond to stimulation with human menopausal gonadotrophin (hMG) or only a poor response? Is it represented by consistently poor quality oocytes or by heterozygosity for X-linked disease?

NOMENCLATURE

Premature ovarian failure may be defined as a high plasma concentration of FSH in a woman under the age of 40 with no demonstrable follicular activity. This condition probably occurs in about 1% of women of reproductive age[1,2] and is important because of its association with premature bone loss and increased risk of coronary atherosclerosis. Ginsburg[3] described 1001 consecutive women under the age of 40 presenting with amenorrhoea at an endocrine clinic; 8% had primary amenorrhoea, 9% had premature ovarian failure and 7% were considered to have resistant ovary syndrome. Because of the uncertain prognosis of these women, some of whom show remission of amenorrhoea and even achieve pregnancy, the designation of premature ovarian failure seems inappropriate and the term hypergonadotrophic hypogonadism[4] has been suggested as a more appropriate alternative.

CAUSES

The distribution of causes of hypergonadotrophic hypogonadism varies from study to study. For example, although immune causes are said to account for 17% of cases[5] (Table 1) this varies from 3% of those presenting with amenorrhoea in 1001 patients[3] to 22 of 57 patients (39%) in a smaller study[6]. Although patients have been classified as having hypergonadotrophic

Table 1 Causes of hypergonadotrophic hypogonadism in 115 patients. (Modified from ref. 4)

Chromosomal	25%
Immune	17%
Chemotherapy, radiation, infection	11%
Idiopathic	47%

Table 2 Comparison of 18 patients with primary hypergonadotrophic amenorrhoea and 97 patients with secondary hypergonadotrophic amenorrhoea

	Primary	*Secondary*
Oestrogen deficiency (%)	22	86
Incomplete sex development (%)	89	8
Chromosomal abnormality (%)	56	13
Pregnant before diagnosis (%)	0	34
Ovulation after diagnosis (%)	0	24
Pregnant after diagnosis (%)	0	8

hypogonadism of genetic, autoimmune or other origin[5], the causes of the condition have been further divided (Table 1). It is striking that virtually half of these patients are characterized as idiopathic.

Rebar and Connolly[4] made a useful comparison of the characteristics of patients with primary and secondary hypergonadotrophic amenorrhoea (Table 2). Their definition encompassed those women with amenorrhoea lasting at least 4 months, with a peripheral serum FSH concentration >40 IU/l (second International Reference Preparation (IRP) hMG). They excluded those with surgical menopause and were restrictive in their age-definition to those under the age of 30. Oestrogen deficiency was much more common in those with secondary amenorrhoea, whereas incomplete development of secondary sexual characteristics was more common in those with primary amenorrhoea. Similarly, chromosomal abnormalities were more common in those with primary amenorrhoea. Ovulatory activity leading to pregnancy was only a feature of those with secondary amenorrhoea, constituting some 17% in the study of Hague and colleagues[6]. Although karyotypes were banded

Table 3   Characteristics of pubertal hypergonadotrophic hypogonadism

Chromosomally incompetent ($n = 69$)	
45X	24
Y cell lines	12
Structural abnormalities of X	25
(isochromosome, others)	
Other mosaic cell lines	8
Chromosomally competent ($n = 40$)	
46, XX	34
46, XY	6

this may not detect some deletions and so was only an approximate indicator of chromosomal abnormality. Reflecting oestrogen deficiency, over half of the cases described had a demonstrable reduction in bone density, whereas those who demonstrated subsequent ovulatory activity tended to have a higher basal plasma oestradiol concentration.

A much earlier study[7], performed before the advent of the more sophisticated molecular biological techniques for analysis of karyotypes, produced a useful classification of a series of patients with pubertal hypergonadotrophic hypogonadism, dividing them into chromosomally incompetent and chromosomally competent (Table 3). A recent study[8] describing FSH β-gene structure used a further classification around the stages of reproductive life. Primary amenorrhoea could be divided into those with delayed puberty or arrested pubertal development whereas secondary premature ovarian failure distinguished the events occurring early (post-pubertal but before reproduction) and late (failure post-reproduction). Deletions on the X chromosome[9] have been correlated with clinical signs. Primary amenorrhoea can be associated with deletions from p11.4 to q26 whereas women with less severe clinical manifestations, such as secondary amenorrhoea or oligomenorrhoea, or even those who have regular menses and are fertile, may have deletions covering a larger area of the short arm of the X chromosome from p2 to 22.1. Curiously, in all patients the most distal parts of the short and long arm of the X chromosome have been spared.

RESISTANT OVARY SYNDROME

Resistant ovary syndrome has always been difficult to distinguish from genuine premature ovarian failure. Although the plasma FSH concentration is high, these patients may respond to very high doses of hMG or FSH. Formerly, ovarian biopsy was recommended as a means of distinguishing women with ovarian follicles unresponsive to stimulation from those showing depletion of follicles. However, it was appreciated that biopsies were not representative, and pregnancies were documented in women whose biopsies had suggested premature ovarian failure. Obtaining a biopsy involves an invasive procedure, although this could be performed laparoscopically. More recently[10], ultrasound has been used in an attempt to discriminate between these patients; however at least one ovary could not be visualized in those of 17 women studied. It was suggested that an absence of follicles in an ovary of small volume indicated true premature ovarian failure. On the other hand, if follicles were present, the ovarian volume was normal and one might expect these individuals to respond to treatment. This hypothesis awaits testing. Another explanation for resistant ovary syndrome[11] is that LH of high molecular weight may not stimulate LH receptors, resulting in a non-functioning ovary.

Treatments that have been used include GnRH down-regulation, plasmaphoresis and immunosuppression, or simply increasing the dose of gonadotrophin administered.

MECHANISMS IN HYPERGONADOTROPHIC HYPOGONADISM

There are several possible causes of hypergonadotrophic hypogonadism. These may be related to FSH production, function of the FSH receptor and signal transduction after ligand binding.

DNA responsible for FSH production could be influenced by genes on the X chromosome at the terminal segment q25, or there could be a defect in the FSH gene itself, which is located on chromosome 11 p13. Although there does not seem to be a major deletion, the existence of a small or point deletion which has not yet been characterized is quite likely. It is possible that aberrant mRNA is produced and has altered translation or degradation rates. It is also possible that a mutation has abolished the codons for glycosylation. There is certainly heterozygosity and polymorphism in the LH β-gene[12] as demonstrated by restriction fragment length polymorphism following digestion with the restriction enzyme *Hind*III. Fragments of 15 kb and 12 kb have been identified, and individuals can show homozygosity for each or heterozygosity, with both fragments expressed. There may also be an alteration in conformation of FSH, resulting in the production of isoforms. The presence of an isoform[11] of FSH in either premature ovarian failure or resistant ovary syndrome may alter signal transduction, a process demonstrated in sheep testes where the isoform contained an altered carboxyl group[13]. The α and β subunits may be free, or structural changes could lead to a lack of binding to the receptor.

There could also be a mutation in the FSH receptor, causing a lack of ligand binding. Examination of exon 10 by the polymerase chain reaction[14] provided evidence of heteroduplex formation on denaturing gel electrophoresis, and a mutation was noted in five of 13 subjects studied. Although circulating immunoglobulin (Ig) has been identified[15,16], Weetman[17] has suggested that detection of this blocking antibody may depend on the purity of the IgG preparation.

The LH receptor has been described by McFarland and colleagues[18]. It was first identified in the pig, following which the FSH receptor was identified in rat Sertoli cells. The two receptors are very similar; hydrophobic analysis reveals seven transmembrane sequences[19]. There is an unusually large extracellular ligand binding domain with repetitive sequences showing significant homology to the leucine-rich glycoprotein family of proteins[20]. The extracellular and intracellular domains contain several potential glycosylation sites, and the intracellular domain also contains potential phosphorylation sites.

It is thought that in the resting state the α and β components of the stimulatory G protein complex are conformationally related to one another and linked to guanidine diphosphate[21]. Activation by ligand binding to the receptor induces a change in conformation and activation of adenylate cyclase. A change in signal transduction from the receptor could be caused by a mutation in one of the G protein constituents α and β, shown to be present in the McCune–Albright syndrome, characterized by precocious puberty, café au lait spots and autonomously functioning ovarian cysts. Melanocyte activation occurs in this syndrome, thought to be due to G protein stimulation without ligand binding. A germ-line mutation has also been described in Albright's hereditary osteodystrophy. These patients are unresponsive to parathyroid and other trophic hormones, suggesting that the stimulatory G protein complex fails to couple the hormone receptor with adenylate cyclase[22]. An inhibitory G protein complex also exists and a reduction in hormonal inhibition of adenylate cyclase mediated by this protein has been shown in growth hormone-secreting pituitary tumours and in some neoplastic thyroid diseases, as well as in type 1 diabetes mellitus. There may also be a defect in cyclic GMP phosphodiesterase which results in prolonged activity of GTP; this has been associated with the retinal degeneration of retinitis pigmentosa. Alternative mutations could occur in the adenylate cyclase binding protein or in the cAMP-dependent protein kinase A.

AUTOIMMUNE OOPHORITIS

Histologically, autoimmune oophoritis has been described as a lympho-cytic and plasma cell infiltrate associated with endocrine hilar cells, theca interna and corpora lutea but not primordial follicles[16]. However, more than half of these cases have no infiltrate. Differential staining for T-cells reveals CD-4 positive cells.

Autoimmune ovarian disease can be a feature of a number of polyendocrine syndromes[16]. Ovarian failure occurs in 17% of patients with type I disease, described as featuring two of Addison's disease, hypoparathyroidism and chronic mucocutaneous candidiasis. Type II comprises Addison's disease, thyroid disease and/or type I diabetes mellitus. Type III is more usually included in type II and features thyroiditis and endocrinopathy other than Addison's disease. Gonadal failure occurs in about 4% of these patients. Altogether, 18% of patients with types I and II autoimmune ovarian failure have associated non–ovarian disease. There is also the rare POEMS syndrome, an acronym for polyneuropathy organomegaly involving the spleen and lymph glands, endocrinopathy, monoclonal gammopathy which is λ-light chain restricted and skin changes characterized by hyperpigmentation and thickening.

Several possible causes of immune activation are thought to occur as a result of tissue damage. Assessment of antibodies present in 40 patients with premature ovarian failure showed that, relative to controls, there was a significant increase in antibodies against thyroglobulin, nuclear antigens, heart tissue and gluten, and increased levels of IgM. In addition, decreased levels of complement components C3 and C4[23] and anti-ooplasm antibodies have also been described[24].

The immune response to ovarian tissue includes steroid cell antibodies as an indication of B-cell response. These are found by cross-reaction in one-quarter of patients with Addison's disease[25]. Luborsky and colleagues, using an enzyme-linked immunosorbent assay, showed cross-reaction between an ovarian homogenate and the Fallopian tube[26].

Peripheral T lymphocytes have also been shown to be activated in autoimmune oophoritis. Expression of the major histocompatibility complex II HLA-DR antigens is increased, and although serum soluble forms were not found, ovarian expression of the 55 kD α-chain interleukin 2-receptor was increased in comparison with controls[27]. An increase in the number of T cells expressing T1 α was noted[28], and although these authors could not demonstrate an increase in T helper/ T suppressor cell ratios (CD4/CD8), this has been disputed, an increase being demonstrated after hormone replacement therapy[29,30].

Recent studies show no specific cross-reaction between sonicated membranes from human ovaries and bovine corpora lutea and auto-immune sera from women with premature ovarian failure, as measured by enzyme-linked immunosorbent assay, although there was significant cross-reaction with Fallopian tube antigens[31]. However, the existence of antibodies to soluble fractions clearly needs to be examined.

In the investigation of hypergonadotrophic hypogonadism, myotonia dystrophica[17] and 17α-hydroxylase deficiency need to be excluded. Galactosaemia has previously been associated with premature ovarian failure, but a recent study of 108 women carrying a deficiency of the enzyme galactose 1-phosphate uridyl transferase (GALT) did not show an increased frequency of premature menopause[32]. The association of blepharophimosis and true premature menopause or resistant ovary syndrome has also been noted[33].

INVESTIGATION

Apart from a systematic history and physical examination, a number of investigations have been recommended[4]. These are: full blood count, erythrocyte sedimentation rate, fasting blood sugar, serum calcium and phosphate, serum protein and albumin/globulin ratio, rheumatoid factor and anti–nuclear antigen, anti–thyroid globulin and anti-microsomal antibodies. The endocrine survey should comprise measurement of serum thyroxine, thyroid stimulating hormone, follicle stimulating hormone, luteinizing hormone and oestradiol. An assessment of adrenal reserve, either by a morning cortisol measurement or synthetic adrenocortico-trophin stimulation, should be undertaken, along with imaging of the sella turcica, an assessment of bone density and karyotyping.

MANAGEMENT

Oestrogen–progestogen combinations

Some patients with amenorrhoea respond to administration of oestrogen or sequential oestrogen/progestogen. A spontaneous pregnancy occurring immediately after an unsuccessful egg donation has been reported[34]. On the other hand, serial weekly measurement of FSH/LH and oestradiol for 5 weeks showed fluctuation in some patients but not in others. Differences in profiles did not predict response to high-dose hMG[35].

Ovulation induction regimens

The most optimistic report[36] was that of treatment by induction of ovulation in 100 patients with hypergonadotrophic hypogonadism. There were eight pregnancies, in patients who had suffered from amenorrhoea for an average of 2.2 years, although this study has been criticized as being uncontrolled. Pregnancy has been reported as long as 14 years after the onset of secondary amenorrhoea[37]. Nelson and co-workers[38] reported a prospective cross-over, randomized controlled trial in which 26 patients were each treated for 4 months with placebo and 4 months with replacement oestradiol on a background of daily subcutaneous administration of gonadotrophin releasing hormone (GnRH) analogue. All patients had normal karyotypes. Four (17%) ovulated, but only after stopping oestradiol hormone replacement. Administration of a GnRH analogue, followed by its withdrawal to induce a rebound phenomenon, was used in eight patients, and compared with treatment using a GnRH analogue and hMG[39]. Ovulation occurred in one patient with each treatment regimen.

Steroid therapy

Steroids have also been used to treat anovulatory patients with autoimmune diseases although the term implied any immune abnormality[23]. Steroids with added hMG resulted in two spontaneous pregnancies (13%) after cessation of ovulation induction. When these patients were down-regulated with GnRH analogue and treated with hMG as well as steroid suppression, 40% of 30 patients conceived. The authors recommended that the treatment should continue for three cycles; if pregnancy was not achieved by that time egg donation should be pursued. Corenblum and colleagues[40] described a regimen of prednisone, 25 mg four times daily for 2 weeks. This was particularly useful in patients with autoimmune thyroiditis whose secondary amenorrhoea due to hypergonadotrophic hypogonadism had lasted <2 years. Two of their 11 patients became pregnant. Those not conceiving were recommended to undergo hormone replacement therapy and oocyte donation.

Oocyte donation

Egg donation has also been suggested for those who respond poorly to *in vitro* fertilization, if they have an adequate endometrial histological response to oestradiol valerate and progesterone[41]. There may ultimately be a greater place for oocyte donation in a wider-ranging group of individuals already identified as having occult ovarian failure[42], in whom menses are still regular but there is already an elevated FSH concentration in the early follicular phase.

Oocyte donation has been well described in patients with hyper-gonadotrophic hypogonadism[43]. Sauer and colleagues treated 31 patients aged between 24 and 44 who had a mean of 4.5 embryos transferred. (No more than three embryos can be legally transferred in the UK under the auspices of the Human Fertilisation and Embryology Authority's Code of Practice.) Their implantation rate was 21.1% and ongoing pregnancies or delivery were reported in 58% of patients and 38% of cycles. Although one neonatal death and one intrauterine death were described the number of mulitple births was not reported. The same group[44] has reported a pregnancy following oocyte donation in a patient with galactosaemia and ovarian failure.

Variations on gamete donation have also been reported. Tubal embryo transfer in 11 patients with premature ovarian failure resulted in nine clinical pregnancies and seven deliveries[45]: four sets of twins and three singletons. Transdermal oestrogen support was associated with three viable pregnancies in the six patients so treated[46].

CONCLUSION

Studies using molecular genetics techniques are likely to throw much light on the mechanisms underlying hypergonadotrophic hypogonadism in the near future. At the same time, gamete donation will become much more widespread, providing a different perspective to the treatment of patients suffering from this condition. Longer-term management with surveillance of immune, bone and cardiovascular problems will also be important to sustain a high quality of life.

Once the patient has accepted her ovarian failure, longer-term management with hormone replacement therapy is important to prevent a reduction in bone mass and the increased cardiovascular risk which would otherwise assume clinical importance.

REFERENCES

1. Aiman, J. and Smentek, C. (1985). Premature ovarian failure. *Obstet. Gynecol.*, **66**, 9–14
2. Coulam, C.B., Adamson, S.C. and Annegers, J.F. (1986). Incidence of premature ovarian failure. *Obstet. Gynecol.*, **67**, 604–6
3. Ginsburg, J. (1991). What determines the age at the menopause? *Br. Med. J.*, **302**, 1288–9
4. Rebar, R.W. and Connolly, H.V. (1990). Clinical features of young women with hypergonadotropic amenorrhea. *Fertil. Steril.*, **53**, 804–10
5. Franks, S. (1991). Diagnosis and treatment of anovulation. In Hillier, S.G. (ed.) *Ovarian Endocrinology*, pp. 226–59. (Oxford: Blackwell Scientific Publications)
6. Hague, W.M., Tan, S.L., Adams, J. and Jacobs, H.S. (1987). Hypergonadotropic amenorrhea–etiology. An outcome in 93 young women. *Int. J. Gynaecol. Obstet.*, **25**, 121–5
7. Reindollar, R.H., Byrd, J.R. and McDonough, P.G. (1981). Delayed sexual development: a study of 252 patients. *Am. J. Obstet. Gynecol.*, **155**, 371–80

8. Layman, L.C., Shelley, M.E., Huey, L.O., Wall, S.W., Tho, S.P.T. and McDonough, P.G. (1993). Follicle-stimulating hormone beta gene structure in premature ovarian failure. *Fertil. Steril.*, **60**, 852–7

9. Simpson, J.L. (1991). Genetic source of femininity. *Fertil Steril.*, **56**, 1206–7

10. Mehta, A.E., Matwijiw, I., Myons, E.A. and Faiman, C. (1992). Non-invasive diagnosis of resistant ovary syndrome by ultrasonography. *Fertil. Steril.*, **57**, 56–61

11. Mason, M., Fonseca, E., Ruiz, J.E., Moran, C. and Zarate, A. (1992). Distribution of follicle-stimulating hormone and luteinizing hormone isoforms in sera from women with primary ovarian failure compared with that of normal reproductive and postmenopausal women. *Fertil. Steril.*, **58**, 60–5

12. Layman, L.C., Reindollar, R.H., Penzias, A.S. and Gray, M.R. (1993). Luteinizing hormone-beta (LH beta) gene DNA sequence differences in women with 46, XX premature ovarian failure. Presented at the *American Fertility Society conjointly with the Canadian Fertility and Andrology Society*, October, Montreal

13. Yarney, T.A., Khan, H., Jiang, L., Macdonald, E.A. and Sairam, M.R. (1993). Detection of a putative isoform of the ovine testicular FSH receptor bearing a variant carboxyl terminus. Presented at the *American Fertility Society conjointly with the Canadian Fertility and Andrology Society*, October, Montreal

14. Whitney, E.A., Su, B.S., Chan, P.C. and Kalugdan, T. (1993). Evidence for mutations in the gene for follicle stimulating hormone receptor (FSH) in women with 46, XX premature ovarian failure by denaturing gradient gel electrophoresis. Presented at the *American Fertility Society conjointly with the Canadian Fertility and Andrology Society*, October, Montreal

15. van Weissenbruch, M.U., Hoek, A., van Vliet-Blecker, I., Schoemaker, J. and Drexhage, H. (1991). Evidence for existence of immunoglobulins that block ovarian granulosa cell growth in vitro. A putative role in resistant ovary syndrome. *J. Clin. Endocrinol. Metab.*, **73**, 360–7

16. Chiauzzi, V., Cigorraga, S., Escobar, M.E., Rivarola, M.A. and Charreau, E.H. (1982). Inhibition of follicle-stimulating hormone receptor binding by circulating immunoglobulins. *J. Clin. Endocrinol. Metab.*, **54**, 1221–8

17. Weetman, A.P. (1991). *Auto-Immune Endocrine Disease*. (Cambridge: Cambridge University Press)

18. McFarland, K.C., Sprengel, R., Phillips, H.S., Kohler, M., Rosemblit, N., Nikolocs, K., Segaloff, D.L. and Seeburg, P.H. (1989). Lutropin-choriogonadotropin receptor: an unusual member of the G-protein-coupled receptor family. *Science*, **245**, 494–9

19. Hillier, S.G. (1991). Cellular basis of follicular endocrine function.

In Hillier, S.G. (ed.) *Ovarian Endocrinology*, pp. 73–106. (Oxford: Blackwell Scientific Publications)

20. Vihko, K.K., LaPolt, P.S., Xiao-Chi, J. and Hsueh, A.J.W. (1991). Regulation of LH and FSH receptor gene expression in the ovary and testes. In Leung, P.C.K., Hsueh, A.J.W. and Friesen, H.G. (eds.) *Molecular Basis of Reproductive Endocrinology*, Serono Symposia, pp. 92–101. (New York: Springer-Verlag)

21. Darnell, J., Lodish, H. and Baltimore, D. (1986). *Molecular Cell Biology* (New York: Scientific American Books)

22. McDonough, P.G. (1992). Editorial comment. *Fertil. Steril.*, **58**, 219–20

23. Bloomenfeld, Z., Halachmi, S., Alik Pretz, B., Shmuel, Z., Golan, D., Makler, A. and Brandes, J.M. (1993). Premature ovarian failure – the prognostic application of auto-immunity on conception after ovulation induction. *Fertil. Steril.*, **59**, 750–5

24. Vallotton, M.B. and Forbes, A.P. (1966). Antibodies to cytoplasm of ova. *Lancet*, **2**, 264–5

25. Irvine, W.J. and Barnes, E.W. (1975). Addison's disease, ovarian failure and hypoparathyroidism. *Clin. Endocrinol. Metab.*, **4**, 379–434

26. Luborsky, J.L., Visintin, I., Boyers, S., Asari, T., Caldwell, B. and DeCherney, A. (1990). Ovarian antibodies detected by immobilised antigen immunoassay in patients with premature ovarian failure. *J. Clin. Endocrinol. Metab.*, **70**, 69–75

27. Nelson, L.M., Kimzey, L.M., Merrian, G.R. and Fleisher, T.A. (1991). Increased peripheral T lymphocyte activation in patients with karyotypically normal spontaneous premature ovarian failure. *Fertil. Steril.*, **55**, 1082–7

28. Rabinowe, E.S.L., Ravnikar, V.A., Dib, S.A., George, K.L. and Dluhy, R.G. (1989). Premature menopause: monoclonal antibody defined T lymphocyte abnormalities and anti-ovarian antibodies. *Fertil. Steril.*, **51**, 450–6

29. Ho, P.C., Tang, G.W.K., Fu, K.H., Fan, M.C. and Lawton, J.W.M. (1988). Immunologic studies in patients with premature ovarian failure. *Obstet. Gynecol.*, **71**, 622–6

30. Ho, P.C., Tang, G.W.K. and Lawton, J.W.M. (1991). Lymphocyte subsets in patients with oestrogen deficiency. *J. Reprod. Immunol.*, **20**, 85–91

31. Wheatcroft, N.J., Toogood, A.A., Li, T.C., Cooke, I.D. and Weetman, A.P. (1994). Detection of antibodies to ovarian antigens in women with premature ovarian failure. *Clin. Exp. Immunol.*, in press

32. Kaufman, F.R., Devgan, S. and Donell, G.M. (1993). Results of a survey of carrier women for the galactosemia gene. *Fertil. Steril.*, **760**, 727–8

33. Fraser, I.S., Shearman, R.P., Smith, A. and Russell, P. (1988). An association among blepharophimosis, resistant ovary syndrome, and true premature menopause. *Fertil. Steril.*, **50**, 747–51

34. Santoro, N. and Schmidt, C.L. (1990). Pregnancy after an unsuccessful oocyte donation cycle. *Fertil. Steril.*, **53**, 174–6

35. Boyers, S.P., Luborsky, J.L. and DeCherney, A.H. (1988). Usefulness of serial measurements of serum follicle stimulating hormone, luteinizing hormone and estradiol in patients with premature ovarian failure. *Fertil. Steril.*, **50**, 408–12

36. Check, J.H., Nowroozi, K., Chase, J.S., Nazari, A., Chapse, D. and Vaze, M. (1990). Ovulation induction and pregnancies in 100 consecutive women with hypergonadotrophic amenorrhea. *Fertil. Steril.*, **53**, 811–16

37. Jacobson, A., Galen, D.I. and Weckstein, L.N. (1991). Reproductive roulette-prognosis for ovarian failure. *Fertil. Steril.*, **55**, 446–7

38. Nelson, L.M., Kimsey, L.M., White, B.J. and Merrian, G.R. (1992). Gonadotropin suppression for the treatment of karyotypically normal spontaneous premature ovarian failure: a controlled trial. *Fertil. Steril.*, **57**, 50–5

39. Rosen, G.F., Stone, S.C. and Yee, B. (1992). Ovulation induction in women with premature ovarian failure: a prospective, cross-over study. *Fertil. Steril.*, **57**, 448–9

40. Corenblum, B., Rowe, T. and Taylor, P.J. (1993). High-dose, short-term glucocorticoids for the treatment of infertility resulting from premature ovarian failure. *Fertil. Steril.*, **59**, 988–91

41. Remohi, J., Vidal and Pellicer, A. (1993). Oocyte donation in low responders to conventional ovarian stimulation for *in vitro* fertilisation. *Fertil. Steril.*, **59**, 1208–15

42. Cameron, I.T., O'Shea, F.C., Rolland, J.M., Hughes, E.G., de Kretzer, D.M. and Healy, D.L. (1988). Occult ovarian failure: a syndrome of infertility, regular menses, and elevated follicle-stimulating hormone concentrations. *J. Clin. Endocrinol. Metab.*, **67**, 1190–4

43. Sauer, M.V., Paulson, R.J., Macaso, T.M., Francis, M.M. and Lobo, R.A. (1991). Oocyte and pre-embryo donation to women with ovarian failure: an extended clinical trial. *Fertil. Steril.*, **55**, 39–43

44. Sauer, M.V., Kaufman, F.R., Paulson, R.J. and Lobo, R.A. (1991). Pregnancy after oocyte donation to a woman with ovarian failure and classical galactosemia. *Fertil. Steril.*, **55**, 1197–9

45. Rotsztjn, D.A., Remohi, J., Weckstein, L.N., Ord, T., Moyer, D.L., Balmaceda, J.P. and Asch, R.H. (1990). Results of tubal embryo transfer in premature ovarian failure. *Fertil. Steril.*, **54**, 348–50

46. Droesch, K., Navot, D., Scott, R., Kreiner, D., Liu, H.-C. and Rosenwaks, Z. (1988). Transdermal estrogen replacement in ovarian failure for ovum donation. *Fertil. Steril.*, **50**, 931–4

9

Hypo-oestrogenism: consequences and management

D. H. Barlow

INTRODUCTION

Many hypothalamic–pituitary disorders result in amenorrhoea and low circulating oestrogen levels since the gonadotrophin stimulus to ovarian activity is defective. Conditions associated with ovarian failure, both congenital and acquired, will produce the same hypo-oestrogenic state. Many of the issues discussed will, therefore, be relevant to these women also, although they are not the focus of the paper. In addition, it is important to emphasize that most of our understanding of the effects of oestrogen deficiency is based on data obtained in women who have undergone the physiological ovarian failure of the menopause.

For many women affected by hypothalamic–pituitary amenorrhoea the priorities are obtaining a diagnosis and then achieving a pregnancy. For others, once a diagnosis of the amenorrhoea has been reached the priority is to deal with the symptoms or chronic physical problems affecting the skeleton or the cardiovascular system as a result of low oestrogen levels. The clinician must also bear in mind other clinical priorities: psychiatric help may be needed when the problem is anorexia nervosa, and measures to ensure adequate physical maturation are required when the problem is congenital and interferes with the processes of puberty.

VASOMOTOR SYMPTOMS

The hypo-oestrogenism of the menopause is well known to be associated with a high prevalence of flushes and sweats: these can cause inconvenience or real distress. While vasomotor symptoms are an extremely common symptom of the menopause they are by no means as common in younger women with hypothalamic–pituitary amenorrhoea. This is not simply an age difference since distressing flushes are a common symptom when young women who do not have a hypothalamic–pituitary problem are treated with gonadotrophin hormone releasing hormone (GnRH) agonist for a chronic indication. There is evidence of autonomic dysfunction in hypothalamic–pituitary amenorrhoea and, since there is autonomic involvement in the flush process, perhaps this link is a factor in the tendency for flushing to be absent in such cases.

Despite the fact that hot flushes and sweats affect most women in the climacteric the underlying mechanisms remain poorly understood. Hot flushes involve a transient rise in skin temperature at a time when core temperature is not elevated[1]. The increased blood flow through the upper body gives rise to heat loss which can be demonstrated by thermography[2]. These events are associated with neuroendocrine events which include LH surges[3]. While involvement of endogenous opiate activity has been suggested[4] the data on this are conflicting[5]. The severity of flushing correlates with aberrant autonomic control of skin blood flow[6].

The lack of a full understanding might relate to the fact that effective treatment is available despite the uncertainty of the precise mechanism. There is no doubt that oestrogen relieves vasomotor symptoms in most women. The data available relate to menopausal women but similar responses are seen in younger women. Coope[7] and colleagues showed that improvement can be achieved with placebo treatment, but that this is less than that achieved with oestrogen. When the two treatment groups crossed over, those previously receiving placebo further improved on oestrogen, but the oestrogen-treated women deteriorated markedly when transferred to placebo treatment[7]. Progestogen is also capable of providing at least some improvement in women with flushes and full relief for some, although the response is less predictable than with oestrogen[8]. Even less consistent is the response to the autonomic agent clonidine, but data from a controlled trial suggest that it will help some women[9].

GENITAL ATROPHY

Sustained hypo-oestrogenism is likely to result in some degree of genital atrophy. Symptoms, if present, may be limited to those associated with mucosal dyspareunia or vaginal dryness, since the shrinkage of organs such as the uterus will not give rise to symptoms. Even after the menopause, when chronic oestrogen deficiency is well established, only a proportion of women actually complain of discomfort, so it must not be assumed that these younger women will have a problem. Little has been written on this aspect of oestrogen deficiency in hypothalamic– pituitary amenorrhoea but in my experience these women rarely complain of such symptoms. However, some young women rendered acutely hypo-oestrogenic by treatment with a GnRH agonist report dyspareunia when asked about symptoms[10].

PSYCHOLOGICAL SYMPTOMS

Even in the climacteric and the postmenopausal state, for which there are reasonable data, there is no consensus concerning a relationship between oestrogen deficiency and psychological dysfunction.

Bungay and co-workers have reported the clustering of some psychological symptoms around the menopausal transition years[11]. These symptoms included lack of confidence and difficulty making decisions. Poor concentration and memory, depressed mood, tiredness and lack of libido have also been reported in oestrogen-deficient women and attributed to oestrogen deficiency. Studies with hormone replacement therapy have suggested an improvement in some of these symptoms on treatment, leading to the conclusion that the symptoms result directly from oestrogen deficiency[12]. An alternative hypothesis is that the psychological symptoms are not a direct result of oestrogen deficiency but are secondary to the effect of vasomotor symptoms and associated insomnia. Studies which fail to demonstrate a significant rise in psychological symptoms in menopausal women can be cited in support of this view as well as data showing a close correlation between improvement in flushes and improvement in these symptoms on therapy[13,14].

Whether or not oestrogen deficiency directly causes significant psychological symptoms, it is recognized that the acute hormonal transitions of the menstrual cycle and perimenopausal ovarian activity do affect mood adversely in some women. High doses of oestrogen, sustained without fluctuation when given subcutaneously by implant or transdermally by patch, appear to help improve mood[15]. We know that oestrogen can affect the activity of neurotransmitters which modulate mood[16]. It is possible that the therapeutic effect of sustained high oestrogen levels on mood is via a pharmacological action on these neurotransmitters, even if the symptoms are not directly due to oestrogen deficiency.

In hypothalamic–pituitary amenorrhoea, psychological symptoms, possibly resulting from oestrogen deficiency, are not common presenting complaints, but a psychological problem may be present as the underlying cause of the hypothalamic dysfunction. The endocrinologist or gynaecologist should be prepared to recognize this where present and to obtain appropriate psychotherapy for these women.

THE SKELETON AND OESTROGEN

The skeletal effects of premature oestrogen deficiency are a major concern because of the effect of the hypo-oestrogenic state on bone mass, a close correlate of osteoporotic fracture risk. As with the other effects of oestrogen deficiency, our understanding of the processes involved comes mainly from data on menopausal and postmenopausal women, but there is an increasing body of data obtained directly from women with hypothalamic–pituitary amenorrhea. The availability of a measurable end-point parameter, bone density, encourages direct study of this chronic process. In the cardiovascular field we can study only surrogate measures, and it is much more difficult to define the overall effect of oestrogen deficiency or therapeutic interventions.

In eumenorrhoeic women we expect a satisfactory peak bone mass to be achieved in adulthood and to be sustained until menopausal oestrogen deficiency intervenes and induces a relatively rapid loss of bone mass for a few years, followed by a slowing of the rate of loss. When chronic amenorrhoea develops in young adulthood there are a number of scenarios. If oestrogen deficiency is present from the teenage years then a woman's potential peak bone mass may not be achieved. If the oestrogen deficiency is not relieved during adulthood she is likely to experience a progressive loss of bone mass over the decades, significant clinical osteoporosis being a likely outcome. If the oestrogen deficiency is relieved by therapy then she should be able to optimize her remaining potential for bone mass prior to eventually experiencing oestrogen withdrawal when older. A woman who has lost significant bone mass before therapy might reach the menopause with an already impaired skeleton. In such cases there is a good argument for attempting to postpone the menopausal effect by continuing oestrogen replacement for several years past the menopause.

Bone turnover and coupling of resorption formation

It is important for clinicians advising women to have a clear understanding of the dynamic processes which control bone mass since they might otherwise have a too simplistic mechanical concept of the effects of oestrogen deficiency and oestrogen replacement.

Skeletal health is maintained by the continuous interplay of the processes of bone resorption, mediated by osteoclasts, and bone formation, mediated by osteoblasts. There are many stimuli for the induction of the remodelling cycle, including fractures or microfractures and increased mechanical loading, as well as less well-defined skeletal maintainence in which the resting osteocyte population may play a monitoring role. At any moment there are millions of discrete sites of bone resorption involving osteoclastic activity. In order to maintain a relatively constant skeleton these must be in balance with the total number of sites of bone formation. This balance is thought to be the result of the direct coupling of the two processes so that the action of an osteoclast in resorbing bone will itself induce an osteoblastic response at the same site to replace the lost bone. The coupling mechanism appears to involve multiple paracrine signals, particularly interleukin-1, from the osteocyte and transforming growth factor-β released from the matrix of the resorbed bone.

The level of bone turnover determines the rate of initiation of resorption sites and, since there is a time-lag before resorption sites are filled by formation of new matrix and mineralization, any factor which increases bone turnover will initially produce a significant acceleration in bone loss for many months before the coupled increase in bone formation re-establishes the balance between the two processes. Oestrogen deficiency is one factor which increases bone turnover: the onset of oestrogen deficiency therefore temporarily triggers a phase of rapid bone loss.

When bone turnover is reduced, as when hormone replacement therapy is given, this effect is reversed. There is a reduction in the initiation of new resorption sites, but for many months the level of bone formation is determined by the previously high level of resorption, so that there is a relative increase in bone mass which will persist for up to a year or longer. These phenomena which occur when bone turnover rates change must be borne in mind when assessing the effects of treatment interventions since any therapy which lowers bone turnover will temporarily increase bone mass. This effect should not be assumed to continue over a prolonged treatment period. Oestrogen deficiency also induces a relative uncoupling of the balance between resorption and formation to favour resorption, possibly via oestrogen-mediated modulation of osteoblast sensitivity to paracrine signals.

The dynamics of the bone density changes which accompany changes in bone turnover are well demonstrated by the clinical model in which eumenorrhoeic women are rendered oestrogen-deficient by means of a GnRH agonist. The significant bone loss during 6 months of a GnRH agonist treatment results from an increase in bone resorption which can be observed using biochemical markers of bone resorption, which rise at this time[17]. After treatment is stopped, oestrogen levels rise and the lost bone mass is usually regained. Again the biochemical markers of bone formation can be monitored: these rise towards the end of the 6-month treatment period and remain elevated beyond the end of treatment when the markers of resorption have returned to baseline[17].

Bone changes in women with hypothalamic–pituitary hypo-oestrogenism

There is now a body of data indicating that these women do experience bone loss. In 1980 Klibanski and colleagues[18] reported decreased bone density in a series of hyperprolactinaemic women. Similarly in 1984 Rigotti and co-workers[19] reported the same effect in women with anorexia nervosa, while Drinkwater and associates[20] found that amenorrhoeic athletes had reduced bone density. This latter group might have expected skeletal benefit from the exercise but this is less important than the effect of the oestrogen deficiency. Marcus and colleagues[21] subsequently showed that although amenorrhoeic athletes had lower bone density than non-athletic eumenorrhoeic women, these atheletes had higher bone density than non-athletic amenorrhoeic women.

It is possible that the oestrogen deficiency associated with exercise-induced amenorrhoea may have a greater effect than in other forms of amenorrhoea since there can be an alteration in the pattern of oestrogen metabolism to favour catechol-oestrogen production[22]. In a recent report, Davies and co-workers[23] reported that an amenorrhoeic group had a mean reduction in bone density of 15% compared with a control group of normally menstruating age-matched women. The bone loss was related to the duration of the amenorrhoea and to the severity of the oestrogen deficiency rather than to the original cause of amenorrhoea.

There is relatively little published information on the effects of treating amenorrhoeic women to prevent osteoporosis. If the original problem can be treated so that the amenorrhoea ceases, as might be the case in amenorrhoea associated with weight loss or exercise, then it is assumed that the return of normal oestrogen levels will help arrest the problem. Where this is not achieved, or not possible, then oestrogen treatment is necessary. Treasure and colleagues[24] demonstrated benefit from oestrogen in an anorexic population, and Klibansky and Greenspan[25] found an increase in bone in an athletic amenorrhoea group given oestrogen. Dramusic and associates also reported a gain in bone mass in a mixed young hypogonadal population given hormone replacement therapy and emphasized the gain in height observed in those who were sexually immature[26].

CARDIOVASCULAR DISEASE

Bone density measurement provides an indication of any deterioration in the skeleton as a consequence of the hypo-oestrogenism. We have no equivalent measure for the cardiovascular consequences of oestrogen deficiency. It is unlikely that we shall have specific data on the clinical end-points of cardiovascular disease in women who have suffered from hypothalamic–pituitary amenorrhoea. Our understanding of the cardiovascular risk in women who experience significant hypo-oestrogenism during the years before the expected time of the natural menopause is based not on the experience of hypothalamic–pituitary amenorrhoea cases, but on the experience of women with a premature menopause or a surgical menopause.

Ischaemic heart disease

The Framingham study[27] compared women in matched age-groups by menopausal status, and found a significantly higher level of ischaemic heart disease in those who were already menopausal in each age-band. Other American data come from two large studies, the Nurses' Study and Lipid Research Clinics Study. The Nurses' Study indicated that bilateral oophorectomy constituted a risk for ischaemic heart disease but that the natural menopause did not[28], while the Lipid Research Clinics Data suggested the both bilateral oophorectomy and the natural menopause were risk factors[29]. Swedish evidence to suggest that an early menopause increases the risk of cardiovascular disease comes from the data that women with ischaemic heart disease have an earlier mean age of menopause[30], but subsequent work from the same group was less conclusive[31]. There is also a considerable amount of epidemiological evidence to suggest that users of hormone replacement therapy are at a lower risk of ischaemic heart disease[32]; this is supported by direct angiographic data[33] and might be the most important benefit of such treatment in terms of the health of postmenopausal women[34]. The effect of addition of progestogen to hormone replacement therapy to protect the endometrium has been a source of debate since the evidence referred to above is based on treatment with oestrogen without progestogen. Recent evidence from a substantial Swedish study has indicated that the reduction in ischaemic heart disease is maintained where progestogen is added[35].

Lipoprotein changes

Space does not permit a detailed discussion of the complex issues relating to cardiovascular risk in women, but the menopause affects lipoprotein metabolism as well as other aspects of cardiovascular function such as blood flow and the vessel wall. The menopause is associated with a rise in low density lipoprotein (LDL) cholesterol and in high density lipoprotein (HDL) cholesterol subfraction 3 (HDL3), and a slight lowering of the HDL2 level, despite no overall change in total HDL. Triglyceride levels are also raised, but since ageing itself has this effect it is more difficult to detect a specific menopausal influence[36]. Current evidence indicates that these changes should raise cardiovascular risk. Hormone replacement therapy reverses most of these lipid changes[37]. When hypothalamic amenorrhoea is exercise-induced there is the additional complication that exercise itself can have a beneficial effect, with a tendency for HDL to rise and LDL to fall. However, when exercise induces amenorrhoea the overall ratio of apolipoproteins is changed in an adverse direction, with a lowering of the apolipoprotein A-1/apolipoprotein B ratio[38].

There is evidence to suggest that oestrogen has a range of positive effects on the cardiovascular system which are not related to lipid changes. Colour Doppler in the uterine[39] and carotid[40] arteries show increased blood flow in women given oestrogen. Animal data also indicate a direct effect of oestrogen on blood vessel relaxation[41].

In the very long term, oestrogen deficiency may also increase the risk of stroke, this being reduced by hormone replacement therapy. However, even in the menopausal population the data relating to this are conflicting, some important studies suggesting a relationship[42,43] and others finding none[44].

MANAGEMENT

The management of hypothalamic–pituitary hypo-oestrogenism will usually involve some form of hormone replacement, but for some patients lifestyle measures can be of benefit. Maintenance of an adequate dietary calcium intake is worthwhile and regular exercise for those who do not exercise is important. When excessive exercise is the problem some women will be prepared to reduce this, while for those who do not wish to, hormonal treatment may be required. Similarly, some women of very low body weight will be amenable to dietary and behavioural treatment but those in whom anorexia nervosa is the problem will require specialized psychiatric care, particularly in view of the potentially poor prognosis for many such women. One study followed up 100 women with anorexia nervosa for a minimum of 4 years and found that although 48 had a good response to treatment and 30 had an intermediate response, 20 had a poor response and two were dead[45].

Treatment considerations

For women who require oestrogen replacement the options are either standard hormone replacement therapy, as designed for use in older women, or the combined oral contraceptive pill. In the postmenopausal population one of the most important considerations in continuing therapy over a prolonged period is the difficulty in maintaining compliance[46]. When planning long-term replacement in these young women the effects of the hormone replacement formulations are supported by the considerable literature relating to older women, whereas the use of oral contraceptives in this way is not well documented. If, however, the woman would be more likely to continue with oral contraception as a treatment, this would be an appropriate option. These women must realize that if there should be spontaneous recovery of their menstrual function then hormone replacement therapy would not prevent a pregnancy. If compliance is proving to be particularly difficult to sustain, bone densitometry may be helpful, if this is available. If the women has already lost significant bone this may well stimulate her to comply with therapy. Asymptomatic women in whom bone density is still above average may decide not to enter into treatment. These women should appreciate that we cannot readily assess the extent of their cardiovascular risk if they remain without oestrogen for a long period. If the only problem is a dislike of menstruation then they might be offered oestrogen replacement regimens which potentially offer amenorrhoea and which have been developed for use in menopausal women[47]; these protect the skeleton for at least 5 years[48]. Another alternative for the future is to consider combining oral oestrogen with a progestogen-bearing intrauterine contraceptive device, since this provides amenorrhoea for many users as well as contraception and avoids systemic progestogenic side-effects[49]. These devices are not available in the UK.

CONCLUSION

Many women with hypothalamic–pituitary amenorrhoea require a diagnosis and treatment to help them achieve pregnancy, but for others the problems to be addressed are those of oestrogen deficiency. The issues are complex but can be resolved using hormone replacement therapy in most women. However, it is important to tailor the care to the needs of the individual woman, particularly if treatment will be required for many years.

REFERENCES

1. Molnar, G.W. (1975). Body temperatures during menopausal hot flashes. *J. Appl. Physiol.*, **38**, 499–503
2. Sturdee, D.W., Wilson, K.A., Pipili, E. and Crocker, A.D. (1978). Physiological aspects of menopausal hot flush. *Br. Med. J.*, **2**, 79–80
3. Meldrum, D.R., Defazio, J.D., Erlik, Y., Lu, J.K., Wolfsen, A.F., Carlson, H.E., Hershman, J.M. and Judd, H.L. (1984). Pituitary hormones during the menopausal hot flash. *Obstet. Gynecol.*, **64**, 752–6
4. Lightman, S.L. and Jacobs, H.S. (1979). Naloxone: non-steroidal treatment for postmenopausal flushing? *Lancet*, **2**, 1071
5. DeFazio, J., Verheugen, C., Chetkowski, R., Nass, T., Judd, H.L. and Meldrum, D.R. (1984). The effects of naloxone on hot flashes and gonado-tropin secretion in postmenopausal women. *J. Clin Endocrinol. Metab.*, **58**, 578–81
6. Rees, M.C. and Barlow, D.H. (1988). Absence of sustained reflex vaso-constriction in women with menopausal flushes. *Hum. Reprod.*, **3**, 823–5
7. Coope, J. (1976). The effect of 'natural' oestrogen replacement therapy on menopausal symptoms. *Postgrad. Med. J.*, **52** (Suppl. 6), 27
8. Paterson, M.E. (1982). A randomized double-blind cross-over trial into the effect of norethisterone on climacteric symptoms and biochemical profiles. *Br. J. Obstet. Gynaecol.*, **89**, 464–72
9. Clayden, J.R., Bell, J.W. and Pollard, P. (1974). Menopausal flushing: double-blind trial of a non-hormonal medication. *Br. Med. J.*, **1**, 409–12
10. Kennedy, S.H., Williams, I.A., Brodribb, J., Barlow, D.H. and Shaw, R.W. (1990). A comparison of nafarelin acetate and danazol in the treatment of endometriosis. *Fertil. Steril.*, **53**, 998–1003
11. Bungay, G.T., Vessey, M.P. and McPherson, C.K. (1980). Study of symptoms in middle-life with special reference to the menopause. *Br. Med. J.*, **281**, 181–3
12. Brincat, M., Magos, A., Studd, J.W., Cardozo, L.D., O'Dowd, T., Wardle, P.J. and Cooper, D. (1984). Subcutaneous hormone implants for the control of climacteric symptoms. A prospective study. *Lancet*, **1**, 16–8
13. Hunter, M.S. (1990). Emotional well-being, sexual behaviour and hormone replacement therapy. *Maturitas*, **12**, 299–314
14. Ballinger, C.B. (1990). Psychiatric aspects of the menopause. *Br. J. Psychiatry*, **156**, 773–87
15. Studd, J., Watson, N. and Henderson, A. (1990). Oestrogen therapy for the menopause. *Br. J. Psychiatry*, **157**, 931–2

16. Best, N.R., Rees, M.P., Barlow, D.H. and Cowen, P.J. (1992). Effect of estradiol implant on noradrenergic function and mood in menopausal subjects. *Psychoneuroendocrinology*, **17**, 87–93
17. Riis, B.J., Christiansen, C., Johansen, J.S. and Jacobson, J. (1990). Is it possible to prevent bone loss in young women treated with luteinizing hormone-releasing hormone agonsits? *J. Clin. Endocrinol. Metab.*, **70**, 920–4
18. Klibanski, A., Neer, R.M., Beitins, I.Z., Ridgway, E.C., Zervas, N.T. and McArthur, J.W. (1980). Decreased bone density in hyperprolactinemic women. *N. Engl. J. Med.*, **303**, 1511–14
19. Rigotti, N.A., Nussbaum, S.R., Herzog, D.B. and Neer, R.M. (1984). Osteoporosis in women with anorexia nervosa. *N. Engl. J. Med.*, **311**, 1601–6
20. Drinkwater, B.L., Nilson, K., Chesnut, C.H., Bremner, W.J., Shainholtz, S. and Southworth, M.B. (1984) Bone mineral content of amenorrheic and eumenorrheic athletes. *N. Engl. J. Med.*, **311**, 277–81
21. Marcus, R., Cann, C., Madvig, P., Minkoff, J., Goddard, M., Bayer, M., Martin, M., Gandiani, L., Haskell, W. and Genant, H. (1985). Menstrual function and bone mass in elite women distance runners. Endocrine and metabolic features. *Ann. Intern. Med.*, **102**, 158–63
22. Snow, R.C., Barbieri, R.L. and Frisch, R.E. (1989). Estrogen 2-hydroxylase oxidation and menstrual function among elite oarswomen. *J. Clin. Endocrinol. Metab.*, **69**, 369–76
23. Davies, M.C., Hall, M.L. and Jacobs, H.S. (1990). Bone mineral loss in young women with amenorrhoea. *Br. Med. J.*, **301**, 790–3
24. Treasure, J.L., Russell, G.F., Fogelman, I. and Murby, B. (1987). Reversible bone loss in anorexia nervosa. *Br. Med. J. Clin. Res.*, **295**, 474–5
25. Klibanski, A. and Greenspan, S.L. (1986). Increase in bone mass after treatment of hyperprolactinemic amenorrhea. *N. Engl. J. Med.*, **315**, 542–6
26. Dramusic, V., McCarthy, T.G., Yang, M. and Ratnam, S.S. (1993). Implications of premature ovarian failure during adolescence and early adulthood. *Proc. 7th Int Congress on the Menopause, Stockholm*, **1**, 50
27. Gordon, T., Kannel, W.B., Hjortland, M.C. and McNamara, P.M. (1978). Menopause and coronary heart disease. The Framingham Study. *Ann. Intern. Med.*, **89**, 157–61
28. Colditz, G.A., Willett, W.C., Stampfer, M.J., Rosner, B., Speizer, F.E. and Hennekens, C.H. (1987). Menopause and the risk of coronary heart disease in women. *N. Engl. J. Med.*, **316**, 1105–10
29. Bush, T.L., Fried, L.P. and Barrett-Connor, E. (1988). Cholesterol, lipo-proteins, and coronary heart disease in women. *Clin. Chem.*, **34**, B60–70
30. Bengtsson, C. and Lindquist, O. (1979). Menopausal effects on risk factors for ischaemic heart disease. *Maturitas*, **1**, 165–70

31. Lapidus, L., Bengtsson, C. and Lindquist, O. (1985). Menopausal age and risk of cardiovascular disease and death. A 12-year follow-up of participants in the population study of women in Gothenburg, Sweden. *Acta Obstet. Gynecol. Scand.*, **130** (Suppl.), 37–41

32. Stampfer, M.J. and Colditz, G.A. (1991). Estrogen replacement therapy and coronary heart disease: a quantitative assessment of the epidemiologic evidence. *Prev. Med.*, **20**, 47–63

33. Sullivan, J.M., Vander-Zwaag, R., Hughes, J.P., Maddock, V., Kroetz, F.W., Ramanathan, K.B. and Mirvis, D.M. (1990). Estrogen replacement and coronary artery disease. Effect on survival in postmenopausal women. *Arch. Intern. Med.*, **150**, 2557–62

34. Daly, E., Roche, M., Barlow, D., Gray, A., McPherson, K. and Vessey, M. (1992). HRT: an analysis of benefits, risks and costs. *Br. Med. Bull.*, **48**, 368–400

35. Falkeborn, M., Persson, I., Adami, H.O., Bergstrom, R., Eaker, E., Lithell, H., Mohsen, R. and Naessen, T. (1992). The risk of acute myocardial infarction after oestrogen and oestrogen–progestogen replacement. *Br. J. Obstet. Gynaecol.*, **99**, 821–8

36. Stevenson, J.C., Crook, D. and Godsland, I.F. (1993). Influence of age and menopause on serum lipid and lipoproteins in healthy women. *Atherosclerosis*, **98**, 83–90

37. Lobo, R.A. (1991). Clinical review 27: Effects of hormonal replacement on lipid and lipoproteins inpostmenopausal women. *J. Clin. Endocrinol. Metab.*, **73**, 925–30

38. Lamon Fava, S., Fisher, E.C., Nelson, M.E., Evans, W.J., Millar, J.S., Ordovas, J.M. and Schaefer, E.J. (1989). Effect of exercise and menstrual cycle status on plasma lipid, low density lipoprotein particle size, and apolipoproteins. *J. Clin. Endocrinol. Metab.*, **68**, 17–21

39. Bourne, T., Hillard, T.C., Whitehead, M.I., Crook, D. and Campbell, S. (1990). Oestrogens, arterial status, and postmenopausal women. *Lancet*, **335**, 1470–1

40. Gangar, K.F., Vyas, S., Whitehead, M.I., Crook, D., Meire, H. and Campbell, S. (1991). Pulsatility index in internal carotid artery in relation to transdermal oestradiol and time since menopause. *Lancet*, **338**, 839–42

41. Jiang, C.W., Sarrel, P.M., Lindsay, D.C., Poole Wilson, P.A. and Collins, P. (1991). Endothelium-independent relaxation of rabbit coronary artery by 17 beta-oestradiol in vitro. *Br. J. Pharmacol.*, **104**, 1033–7

42. Paganini-Hill, A., Ross, R.K. and Henderson, B.E. (1988). Postmenopausal oestrogen treatment and stoke: a prospective study. *Br. Med. J.*, **297**, 519–22

43. Finucane, F.F., Madans, J.H., Bush, T.L., Wolf, P.H. and Kleinmann, J.C. (1993). Decreased risk of stroke among postmenopausal hormone users. Results from a national cohort. *Arch. Intern. Med.*, **153**, 73–9

44. Stampfer, M.J., Colditz, G.A., Willett, W.C., Manson, J.E., Rosner, B., Speizer, F.E. and Hennekens, C.H. (1991). Postmenopausal estrogen therapy and cardiovascular disease: ten-year follow-up from the Nurses' Health Study. *N. Engl. J. Med.*, **325**, 756–62

45. Hsu, L.K., Crisp, A.H. and Harding, B. (1979). Outcome of anorexia nervosa. *Lancet*, **1**, 61–5

46. Ravnikar, V.A. (1987). Compliance with hormone therapy. *Am. J. Obstet. Gynecol.*, **156**, 1332–4

47. Magos, A.L., Brincat, M., Studd, J.W., Wardle, P., Schlesinger, P. and O'Dowd, T. (1985). Amenorrhea and endometrial atrophy with continuous oral estrogen and progestogen therapy in postmenopausal women. *Obstet. Gynecol.*, **65**, 496–9

48. Christiansen, C. and Riis, B.J. (1990). Five years with continuous combined oestrogen/progestogen therapy. Effects on calcium metabolism, lipoproteins, and bleeding pattern. *Br. J. Obstet. Gynaecol.*, **97**, 1087–92

49. Andersson, K., Mattsson, L.A., Rybo, G. and Stadberg, E. (1992). Intrauterine release of levonorgestrel – a new way of adding progestogen in hormone replacement therapy. *Obstet. Gynecol.*, **79**, 963–7

Index

119